Teaching Exercise to Children

The complete guide to theory and practice

Morc Coulson

Note
Whilst every effort has been made to ensure that the content of this book is as technically accurate and as sound as possible, neither the author nor the publishers can accept responsibility for any injury or loss sustained as a result of the use of this material.

Published by A&C Black Publishers Ltd
36 Soho Square, London W1D 3QY
www.acblack.com

ISBN 978 1 4081 1563 3

A CIP catalogue record for this book is available from the British Library.

Acknowledgements
Cover photograph © www.istockphoto.com
Inside photographs by Joanne Miller
Illustrations by Jeff Edwards
Designed by James Watson

This book is produced using paper that is made from wood grown in managed, sustainable forests. It is natural, renewable and recyclable. The logging and manufacturing processes conform to the environmental regulations of the country of origin.

Typeset in 12.5pt on 10pt URWGroteskTLig by Palimpsest Book Production Limited, Grangemouth, Stirlingshire

Printed and bound in England by Martins The Printers

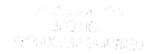

Contents

Foreword by Liz McColgan

Like many other sports in the UK, and especially at grass-roots level, athletics relies on coaches and volunteers to enthuse children of all ages. If delivered in a structured and organised way, sport, athletics and other forms of physical activity can offer children many benefits and rewards. Taking part in sport and exercise can even lead to a possible career, as it did for me, first as a high-level athlete and now as a business woman and coach.

Teaching Exercise to Children offers a comprehensive guide to theoretical knowledge about children and their development, as well as practical applications to help you to shape this development. The book should provide a valuable tool for coaches, teachers, leaders and parents to help them to establish not only the stars of the future but also to cultivate an environment in which sport and exercise can be fun for kids.

Liz McColgan: Mother of five, Olympic Silver medal (10,000 metres), 2 times Commonwealth Gold medal (10,000 metres), World Championship Gold medal (10,000 metres), Commonwealth Bronze medal (3,000 metres), British 10,000 metres record holder, World Cross-country Silver and Bronze medal, World Indoor Silver medal (3,000 metres), Winner of the London and New York Marathons, BBC Sports Personality of the Year.

Acknowledgements

Many thanks to Lucy Beevor, senior editor at A&C Black, who always manages this process professionally and supportively. To my wife Lorretta who understands the time and dedication required but keeps a smile on my face throughout. Finally to my Dad – once again you are, and always will be, my guide.

CHAPTER ONE

Introduction to children and exercise

Objectives

After completing this chapter the reader should be able to:

- Define common terms related to physical activity and exercise.
- Discuss the relationship between these terms.
- Explain the meaning of 'overweight' and 'obese'.
- Identify problems associated with obesity and how they relate to children.
- Discuss statistics in relation to numbers of overweight and obese adults and children.
- Describe activity levels of children in the UK.
- List the health benefits related to physical activity during childhood.
- Understand general and specific guidelines relating to physical activity for children.
- Discuss the topic relating to children and their attitudes to exercise.

Introduction

Before exploring the complex subject of teaching exercise to children (or coaching, as we will refer to it throughout this book), it would be useful to try to gain an understanding of some of the terms that are commonly used within the coaching environment, as sometimes different terms are used by different people to mean the same thing. The descriptions of the terms as outlined in table 1.1 are all adapted from a variety of different sources to try to make them as simple to understand as possible.

Table 1.1 Descriptions of common terms	
Term	**Description**
Physical activity	This term relates to any bodily movement that is produced by the contraction of muscles and that substantially increases the use of energy. Take gardening for instance. Digging soil would require an increase in energy to be able to produce the muscular contraction required.

Physical fitness	This would be the level of ability or abilities that someone would have to help them to perform physical activity. For instance, a certain amount of strength and flexibility is needed to be able to dig.
Exercise (training)	This is the term normally associated with leisure time physical activity conducted with the intention of developing physical fitness. For example, people go to the gym to exercise.
Leisure activity	Leisure activity is often used to describe physical activity undertaken during someone's free time such as golf or rambling.
Health	Health can be described as a state of being free from disease and illness and according to the World Health Organisation it would also include a component of wellness.
Wellness	This not-so common term relates to a state of positive health in the individual which is demonstrated by quality of life and a sense of well-being.

It can be confusing to the reader when some of these common terms are used interchangeably (and sometimes even within the same sentence); to help overcome this, figure 1.1 shows how our own lifestyle and genetics can relate to each of these terms (and also how some of the terms can affect each other). For the purpose of this book, however, we will try to use the term 'activity' (when referring to any form of physical activity or exercise) as a generic blanket term as much as is feasibly possible in order to avoid any potential confusion.

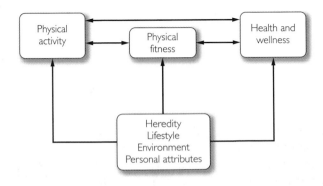

Fig. 1.1 Relationship between physical activity, physical fitness, health and well-being (adapted from Bouchard et al. 1990)

A brief history

Movement, in whatever form, has been an essential part of our development and lifestyle for many thousands of years, ranging from hunting, gathering and fighting for the purpose of survival to well-documented games organised by the likes of the Greeks and the Romans. Whatever the specific purpose of the movement, muscular contraction (work, as we will refer to it for exercise purposes) was needed and hence energy was used in order to do this work. In other words, for many thousands of years we have been a very active species, constantly doing 'work' either for survival or for play.

It could be argued that in recent times we have been hampered somewhat by the advance of technology in the so-called 'modern society'. It wouldn't be difficult to argue that, with the arrival of sedentary pastimes such as computer games, DVDs and internet browsing, this advance does little to help develop future Olympians. Adding this to the problem that we don't need to hunt or gather for survival any more means that we are not as active as we perhaps once were. There is substantial evidence to show that there are many potential benefits for children who do regular physical activity from a participation perspective as well as from a performance perspective. One of the main reasons the government appears to be actively involved in promoting activities for children is because of the alarming rise in numbers of overweight and obese children over the last few decades. As the link between childhood obesity and adult health conditions is well documented, there are concerns that in future this could put an enormous strain on the already overburdened National Health Service (NHS), which the government provides.

Obesity in childhood

The terms 'obesity' and 'overweight' are commonly employed (not just for children), and in many cases are used to mean the same thing; however, they have very different meanings. As precise definitions would be difficult to agree upon, we will take those from the American College of Sports Medicine (ACSM), who have stated the following:

'Overweight' is defined as;
> 'A body weight that exceeds the normal or standard weight for a particular person based on height and frame size'.

'Obesity' is defined as;
> 'Having an excess amount of body fat. For adults in particular, it has been established that men and women with greater than 30% body fat should be considered obese'.

The World Health Organisation (WHO) does not have individual definitions to identify those who are overweight and obese – they use the same definition for both terms;
> 'Overweight and obesity are conditions whereby abnormal or excessive adipose tissue accumulation seriously impairs and endangers health'.

Regardless of the definition of either term, it is clear that someone who is classified as overweight or obese would be considered to have a considerable health risk. It is quite incredible that the British Medical Association (BMA) stated in 2007 that worldwide there were over 22 million children under the age of five years who were severely overweight. In the UK, however, there are around 1 million obese children under 16 years of age, according to the NHS's statistics on obesity. It is thought that these soaring obesity levels have led to an increase in conditions such as childhood type 2 diabetes and will lead to an increase in cases of heart disease, osteoarthritis and some cancers in the future (in fact this is happening already). In terms of looking at the difference between boys and girls and different age ranges, there are many different sources from which to get figures relating to the number of overweight and obese children in the UK population. According to one source, the NHS's statistics on obesity, the change in the proportion of obese children between the ages of 2 and 15 years in the 10-year period 1995–2005 was as follows:

● Boys: A rise from 10.9% to 18.0%
● Girls: A rise from 12.0% to 18.1%

If we look at figures for older children the situation appears to be even worse. For the same 10-year period 1995–2005, and for children between the ages of 11 and 15 years, the figures were as follows:

● Boys: A rise from 13.5% to 20.5%
● Girls: A rise from 15.4% to 20.6%

Did you know
In 2005 almost 871,000 prescriptions items were dispensed in the treatment of obesity, compared with just over 127,000 prescriptions in 1999.

As mentioned previously, not only has obesity risen dramatically over the years but there has also been an alarming increase in childhood type 2 diabetes. One of the most shocking statements by the NHS in 2006 was that it estimates that at least one-fifth of boys and one-third of girls will be obese by the year 2020 if obesity levels continue to rise at the current rate. It is really important to understand that, while children are relatively free of disease and have extremely low mortality rates, it is possible that problems which start during childhood as a result of obesity and diabetes will become chronic diseases in adulthood. In other words, we shouldn't be too complacent about obesity levels in children just because we don't see the complications until they are adults; as figures show, worldwide there are over 1.6 billion (yes, billion!) adults who are overweight and by the year 2015 there will be 2.5 billion adults in the category of overweight or above. This is a major problem because nearly all obese people develop some physical symptoms by the time they are 40, and the majority of these people require some sort of medical assistance for diseases that occur as a direct result of their obesity by the time they are 60. The potential strain on the NHS as a result of this goes without saying.

Did you know

In the UK there are around one million obese children under 16 years of age. That is enough to fill Wembley Stadium more than 10 times!

Why is this increasingly worrying situation such an issue to us as coaches or educators of children, you may ask? Well, according to the Department of Health (DH), obesity reduces life expectancy by an average of nine years (that is a long period in anyone's lifetime), and is directly responsible for over 9000 premature deaths every year. This means that if obesity levels continue to rise at the current rate, many children will actually have a shorter life expectancy than their parents. I think that every coach of children would agree that this is a shocking and almost unbelievable situation for the nation to be in. Fortunately, coaches are in a position to improve or impact on this situation by engaging children in exercise or activity, a responsibility that most would readily accept.

Activity levels

The topic relating to the causes of obesity can be an extremely controversial and delicate one. It has been suggested that some individuals are more genetically susceptible than others to obesity; however, research argues that the recent rapid increase in obesity and overweight levels has occurred over a time period too short for genetic change to be the common cause. In other words, we are told that we shouldn't blame our genes. It has also been suggested that a simpler explanation is that the direct cause of obesity and being overweight is an excess of energy intake over energy expenditure. Put another way, we are guilty of eating too much and exercising too little.

Whether this simplistic view is the case or not, recent figures on children and activity levels have shown a decrease in both the numbers of children participating in activities and the time spent doing them. In 2005 the DH published a report which showed that children now tend to walk or cycle less and less and increasingly rely on cars for transportation. They have also said that children are now tending to opt out of active leisure pursuits and recreational sports and are choosing sedentary entertainment, including television, video games and computers, instead. Research, undertaken by the

Health Education Authority (HEA) in 2007, on leisure time activity showed that approximately 75% of the 11- to 16-year-old children in the UK watched television for two hours per day, and the remainder watched in excess of four hours per day. Their research also showed that computers, computer games and other alternative media activities take up a large proportion of sedentary behaviour, with around 10% of 11- to 16-year-olds playing computer games for in excess of 10 hours per week. Some other interesting figures and statements that came out of the research are as follows:

- Children expend approximately 600kcal (it can take up to an hour to burn this much) per day less than children 50 years ago.
- Since the mid-1980s the average number of miles walked per year has fallen by over 20%.
- Since the mid-1980s the average number of miles cycled has decreased by more than 10%.
- Since the mid-1980s the number of children travelling to school by car has doubled.
- In 2006 only 70% of boys and 59% of girls achieved daily recommended activity levels.

The DH, as well as publishing these kinds of statement, have also stated that physical activity has a significant role to play in contributing to the health and well-being of communities. They have argued that regular exercise and physical activity provide substantial benefits and reduce the risk of developing obesity and all the potential accompanying health defects caused (or made worse) by the disease.

Did you know

In 1998 the government suspended physical education for a period of two years by statutory order for the curriculum of primary schools (ages 5–11). A national survey (Speednet 1999) found that due to this order more than 500,000 hours of physical education was omitted from primary schools throughout England and Wales to make extra time available for literacy and numeracy.

Benefits of activity

Over the years, much research has been done in relation to physical activity and the effects on obesity and especially on the health benefits associated with a physically active lifestyle in children. Figure 1.2 shows just some of these health benefits.

Research also shows that physically active people have a 20–30% reduced risk of premature death and up to a 50% reduced risk of major chronic disease, such as heart disease, stroke, diabetes and cancer, compared to those with a sedentary lifestyle. In fact, it has been suggested that regular participation in physical activity can reduce the risk of developing type 2 diabetes by up to 64% in those at high risk of developing the disease.

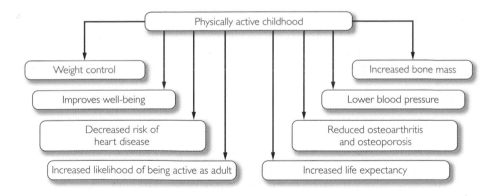

Fig. 1.2 Health benefits associated with a physically active lifestyle

Whether or not this decline in activity and increase in sedentary behaviour has been fully accepted as the main cause of obesity, it is generally recognised that activity for children should be actively promoted so that levels of participation in a variety of activities increase substantially. We do know that doing any kind of activity requires the body to expend energy, so it makes sense to keep children active as much as possible. In view of the alarming obesity statistics there are many guidelines, from various sources, regarding forms of exercise or activity that are thought to help in some way to reduce or impact upon these figures. Even though issues such as nutrition and family involvement are also crucial to this, for the purpose of this book we will concentrate on the area of physical activity only.

General guidelines

It could be said that many young children enjoy being active; however, as parents or as a society, we are often guilty of not providing the opportunity for this to be a regular occurrence. Activities that children prefer tend to be of an interval nature rather than a continuous aerobic nature: in other words, they prefer activities that have short bursts of high intensity followed by longer periods of lower intensity (*see* chapter 4).

It is difficult to agree on the best type of activity to recommend for children because of the many differences such as physical and mental maturity, medical status, skill level and prior experience. It is generally accepted, however, that experiences in childhood are important in terms of the effect on adult participation in activities, so efforts should be made by all coaches to provide positive and enjoyable experiences for children. In other words, adults tend to continue with activities they did as a child. It is also important that children should be educated on the benefits that taking part in various activities can provide (*see* later chapters). This relates not only to benefits at the present time, but also to benefits in the future as a result of regular participation in activities. There are, however, certain institutions and organisations that publish information relating to children and general recommended exercise guidance. In order to simplify this, table 1.2 gives a summary of published guidelines from various organisations and individuals. Note that one of the organisations, the American College of Sports Medicine, is widely regarded as very credible and many of the guidelines in this country are taken from their recommendations.

As you can see from table 1.2, these guidelines are only very general. There are also many other sources of guidelines that are more specific in the types of activity that they recommend. The range also highlights the difference in focus, as some guidelines are related to physical activity only, whereas there are others that acknowledge the importance of including dietary advice as well. For example, The National Institute for Health and Clinical Excellence (NICE) is an independent organisation responsible for providing guidance on promoting good health and on preventing and treating ill health.

Table 1.2 General exercise and activity guidelines

Source	Guidelines
National Institute for Health and Clinical Excellence (2006)	All young people should participate in physical activity of moderate to vigorous intensity for at least one hour a day.
Chief Medical Officer (2004)	Children and young people should achieve a total of a minimum of 60 minutes of at least moderate intensity physical activity each day, and, at least twice a week, include activities to improve muscular strength, flexibility and bone health.
ACSM (2006)	Children should accumulate at least 60 minutes, and up to several hours, of age-appropriate physical activities on all or most days of the week. This should include moderate to vigorous intermittent exercise.
British Association of Sport and Exercise Sciences (BASES) (2006)	At least twice a week young people should carry out activities to help enhance and maintain muscular strength, flexibility and bone health.
Journal of Sports Science 2004 (volume 10)	All young people should be encouraged to participate in safe and effective resistance exercise at least twice a week as part of a balanced exercise and physical education programme.

Table 1.3 NICE guidelines for diet and activity for children	
Diet	• Children and young adults should eat regular meals, including breakfast, in a pleasant, sociable environment, without distractions such as watching television • Parents and carers should eat with children, with all family members eating the same foods
Activity	• Encourage active play – for example dancing and skipping • Try to be more active as a family – for example walking and cycling to school and shops or going to the park or swimming • Gradually reduce sedentary activities such as watching television or playing video games and consider active alternatives such as dance, football or walking • Encourage children to participate in sport or other active recreation, and make the most of opportunities to exercise at school

Table 1.3 gives an outline of some of the guidelines published by NICE in 2006 relating to activities and diet for helping children and young people maintain or work towards a healthy weight.

Even though it is easy to see that the guidelines differ somewhat depending on the source of information, the overall message remains consistent and simple.

Regardless of whatever strategies are used to combat childhood obesity, all sources agree that an increase in activity levels for all children throughout the UK is needed. One of the strategies to mention here is the 'school sport strategy', which was introduced by the UK government in order to increase the take-up of sporting opportunities by 5 to 16 year olds. Essentially the strategy was developed to try to increase the percentage of school children who spent a minimum of two hours each week on high-quality physical education and school sport, within and beyond the curriculum (extended schools and after-school clubs), from 25% in 2002 to 75% by 2006 and to 85% by 2008, and to then increase to a minimum of five hours each week from September 2008. I think those of us who have current experience of school sports, or have witnessed the massive reduction in school sports playing fields over the years, would debate whether or not this target has been achieved, or ever will be in the near future, without a great deal of work at grass-roots level.

Physical education in schools

Much research has been done in relation to children's attitudes towards exercise (in particular to physical education, or PE, at school). It is quite evident from this research that, for whatever reason, not all children enjoy participating in physical education. According to a researcher called Harris, those children who think that they are physically capable or competent are more likely to participate in activities that are of any benefit to health.

Did you know

Over the years, research has consistently shown that one of the main reasons that children participate in activities is *fun*!

Harris also said that those children who avoid sport say the main reason is that they feel they are not good enough to play. This is a widespread problem, as physical education, which for many children is the only form of physical activity they participate in, has been reported to be dominated by competitive team games (sport). In other words, a lot of children do not like the competition element of physical education. It is often reported that about half of children interviewed liked the competition element, whereas about half didn't. All too often, children are put in a position where they are pressurised to 'perform' in front of their friends, or they are left to the end due to 'team-choosing' by more 'able' children. Therefore, it is important that when teaching exercise to children, the coach caters for all levels of ability by allowing children to participate in a range of activities that focus on fun and on a variety of skills, while de-emphasising the competitive aspect of the activity. For this reason, the promotion of non-competitive, fun and enjoyable alternative activities to typical physical education lessons should be provided for those children who do not enjoy the competitive element of sport. In these activities the primary objective should be to increase confidence and self-esteem by focusing on fun and enjoyment.

Other important benefits of non-competitive activities include developing empathy and team skills as well as learning the importance of these types of activity. In other words, the coach should attempt to get the message across that not all activities have to be competitive, and they should attempt to encourage children just to try to participate. It could be argued, therefore, that physical education is the most logical and practical environment in which to promote fun and varied activities to young people, because around 96% of youths are required to take some form of physical education at school.

The National Curriculum for PE

The National Curriculum for PE sets out these comprehensive guidelines in a progressive form by giving a range of units that each school can choose from (for example dance, games or athletic activities), with a range of objectives developed within each unit. These units become more progressive (in terms of complexity and difficulty level) throughout the school key stages. Also, within each of these units are targets that the school should be encouraging and helping children to aim for. These are known as 'attainment targets' and consist of statements about the knowledge, skills and understanding that pupils of different abilities and maturities are expected to have by the end of each key stage (1 to 4). Attainment targets consist of eight levels of increasing difficulty, in addition to which there is a level of exceptional performance, which is above level 8 and the highest level a child can achieve. Each of the levels has a descriptor explaining the type and range of performance that pupils working at that level should characteristically demonstrate, taken from the National Curriculum for PE.

LEVEL 1
Pupils copy, repeat and explore simple skills and actions with basic control and coordination. They start to link these skills and actions in ways that suit the activities. They describe and comment on their own and others' actions. They talk about how to exercise safely, and how their bodies feel during an activity.

LEVEL 2
Pupils explore simple skills. They copy, remember, repeat and explore simple actions with control and coordination. They vary skills, actions and ideas and link these in ways that suit the activities. They begin to show some understanding of simple tactics and basic compositional ideas. They talk about differences between their own and others' performance and suggest improvements. They understand how to exercise safely, and describe how their bodies feel during different activities.

LEVEL 3
Pupils select and use skills, actions and ideas appropriately, applying them with co-ordination and control. They show that they understand tactics and composition by starting to vary how they respond. They can see how their work is similar to and different from others' work, and use this understanding to improve their own performance. They give reasons why warming up before an activity is important, and why physical activity is good for their health.

LEVEL 4
Pupils link skills, techniques and ideas and apply them accurately and appropriately. Their performance shows precision, control and fluency, and they understand tactics and composition. They compare and comment on skills, techniques and ideas used in their own and others' work, and use this understanding to improve their performance. They explain and apply basic safety principles in preparing for exercise. They describe what effects exercise has on their bodies, and how it is valuable to their fitness and health.

LEVEL 5
Pupils select and combine their skills, techniques and ideas and apply them accurately and appropriately, consistently showing precision, control and fluency. When performing,

they draw on what they know about strategy, tactics and composition. They analyse and comment on skills and techniques and how these are applied in their own and others' work. They modify and refine skills and techniques to improve their performance. They explain how the body reacts during different types of exercise, and warm up and cool down in ways that suit the activity. They explain why regular, safe exercise is good for their fitness and health.

LEVEL 6

Pupils select and combine skills, techniques and ideas. They apply them in ways that suit the activity, with consistent precision, control and fluency. When planning their own and others' work, and carrying out their own work, they draw on what they know about strategy, tactics and composition in response to changing circumstances, and what they know about their own and others' strengths and weaknesses. They analyse and comment on how skills, techniques and ideas have been used in their own and others' work, and on compositional and other aspects of performance, and suggest ways to improve. They explain how to prepare for, and recover from, the activities. They explain how different types of exercise contribute to their fitness and health and describe how they might get involved in other types of activity and exercise.

LEVEL 7

Pupils select and combine advanced skills, techniques and ideas, adapting them accurately and appropriately to the demands of the activities. They consistently show precision, control, fluency and originality. Drawing on what they know of the principles of advanced tactics and compositional ideas, they apply these in their own and others' work. They modify them in response to changing circumstances and other performers. They analyse and comment on their own and others' work as individuals and team members, showing that they understand how skills, tactics or composition and fitness relate to the quality of the performance. They plan ways to improve their own and others' performance. They explain the principles of practice and training, and apply them effectively. They explain the benefits of regular, planned activity on health and fitness and plan their own appropriate exercise and activity programme.

LEVEL 8

Pupils consistently distinguish and apply advanced skills, techniques and ideas, consistently showing high standards of precision, control, fluency and originality. Drawing on what they know of the principles of advanced tactics or composition, they apply these principles with proficiency and flair in their own and others' work. They adapt it appropriately in response to changing circumstances and other performers. They evaluate their own and others' work, showing that they understand the impact of skills, strategy and tactics or composition, and fitness on the quality and effectiveness of performance. They plan ways in which their own and others' performance could be improved. They create action plans and ways of monitoring improvement. They use their knowledge of health and fitness to plan and evaluate their own and others' exercise and activity programme.

EXCEPTIONAL PERFORMANCE

Pupils consistently use advanced skills, techniques and ideas with precision and fluency. Drawing on what they know of the principles of advanced strategies and tactics or composition, they consistently apply these principles with originality, proficiency and flair in their own and others' work. They evaluate their own and others' work, showing that they understand how skills, strategy and tactics or composition, and fitness relate to and affect the quality and originality of performance. They reach judgements independently about how their own and others' performance could be improved, prioritising aspects for further development. They consistently apply appropriate knowledge and understanding of health and fitness in all aspects of their work.

National curriculum guidelines

It is difficult for schools to try to facilitate and guide all individual children to achieve the highest attainment level they possibly can, and the range of abilities within any school group is usually vast: therefore, general target ranges are normally set, with a suggested minimum level for the end of key stages. For instance, the majority of pupils are expected to work at the ranges and levels outlined in table 1.4.

Table 1.4 Target ranges for key stages

Key stage	Level range	End stage level
1	1–3	2
2	2–5	4
3	3–7	5/6

Obviously, there will be some children who will exceed these targets and some who will fall short of the targets but, overall, most children will usually fall within the recommended target ranges. It should be remembered, therefore, that the National Curriculum for PE is a set of guidelines that is there for children to aspire to. As mentioned earlier, there are various units that schools can choose to deliver. One of the units that is relevant to some of the 'multi-skills' activities described later (*see* chapter 8) is a unit called 'athletic activities'. Within this unit there are suggested activities and outcomes that are applicable to each key stage (only key stages 1 and 2 are dealt with here). You will see from the athletic activities unit descriptor (taken from the National Curriculum Qualifications and Curriculum Development Agency, www.qcda.gov.uk) that many of the activities and outcomes are met by the multi-skill activities outlined in chapter 8. Within the unit descriptor, there are also a number of key points and health and safety statements. The key points are just general guidelines that help with the delivery of the sessions; the health and safety points that are provided help teachers to keep children (and themselves) as safe as possible throughout the activity programmes.

Unit descriptor – Athletic activities (1) – Key stages 1 and 2

Section 1: Acquiring and developing skills
Objectives – Children should learn:

- to remember, repeat and link combinations of actions
- to use their bodies and a variety of equipment with greater control and coordination

Table 1.1 Activities
1.1 Ask the children to jog in a marked area, around markers, hoops or cones, avoiding contact with each other. Help them to move more freely within the space, anticipating where it is safe to move quickly.
1.2 Ask the children to play follow my leader and change the way they move when they pass a coloured marker, e.g. hop, then jog, then walk backwards, then skip.
1.3 Teach the children to run and turn quickly, and to follow different pathways or tracks.
1.4 Teach them different ways of throwing, e.g. left-handed, right-handed, two-handed, under-arm, over-arm. Help them to throw further and with greater accuracy.
1.5 Teach the children different ways of jumping, e.g. one foot to the other foot (step), two feet to two feet, one foot to the same foot (hop), one foot to two feet, two feet to one foot. Teach them to link some jumps together.
Outcomes
1.6 Demonstrate the five basic jumps on their own, e.g. a series of hops, and in combination, e.g. hop, one-two, two-two, showing control at take-off and landing.
1.7 Run continuously for about one minute and, when required, show the difference between running at speed and jogging.
1.8 Throw with increasing accuracy and coordination into targets set at different distances.
1.9 Demonstrate a range of throwing actions using a variety of games equipment.

Section 2: Selecting and applying skills, tactics and compositional ideas

Objectives – Children should learn:

● to choose skills and equipment to help them meet the challenges they are set

Table 1.2 Activities
2.1 Teach the children to challenge themselves in throwing activities, e.g. by increasing the distance thrown, or by throwing equipment into more difficult targets. Help them to choose the best way of throwing to succeed in the challenge, e.g. under-arm, over-arm, low, high.
2.2 Teach the children to jump and land with control, using different jumps. Help them to understand the difference between jumping high and jumping long.
2.3 Teach them how to choose a speed for running or travelling that suits the task, e.g. more slowly over longer times and distances, more quickly over shorter times and distances. Help them to explain how they have to perform to meet the challenge they have been set, e.g. I need to go fast, I have to be careful.
Outcomes
2.4 Use different techniques, speeds and effort to meet challenges set for running, jumping and throwing.

Section 3: Knowledge and understanding of fitness and health

Objectives – Children should learn:

● to recognise and describe what their bodies feel like during different types of activity

Table 1.3 Activities
3.1 Ask the children to listen to others breathing after exercise.
3.2 Listen to them describe how they feel when they have worked hard. Find out whether they can say when they feel hot, their heart beats fast or they breathe fast.
3.3 Talk to them about how some activities make them feel different from others.

Table 1.3 Outcomes

3.4 Describe what happens to their heart, breathing and temperature during different types of athletic activity.

Section 4: Evaluating and improving performance

Objectives – Children should learn:

● to watch, copy and describe what they and others have done

Table 1.4 Activities

4.1 Teach the children to watch others and to pick out things they do when running, e.g. fast or slow, taking big or small steps, jumping, e.g. hopping, stepping, two feet to two feet, and throwing, e.g. high, low, under-arm, over-arm.

4.2 Listen to the children describe different running speeds and different throwing and jumping actions. Talk to them about how successful they have been. Find out whether they can recognise when they have improved.

Outcomes

4.3 Identify and describe different running, jumping and throwing actions.

4.4 Explain what is successful and what they have to do to perform better.

Key points; Health and safety

Table 1.5 Key points

KP1 In every lesson, most of the children's learning should take place through physical activity relating to the core tasks.

KP2 Most lessons should start with short warm-up activities that help the children remember what they did in the last lesson and prepare them for what they will learn next. Most lessons should end with cool-down activities.

Table 1.5 Key points (cont.)

KP3 Give the children opportunities and time to investigate, explore and practise on their own and with a partner. They should also have opportunities to challenge and measure themselves, and to record some of what they achieve.

KP4 Make sure the children take part in some vigorous activity, so that they can identify how their body changes as a result of exercise.

KP5 Give the children specific guidance on what to do and how to do it, as well as general feedback and praise.

Health and safety

HS1 Do the children's clothing and footwear help their learning and keep them safe?

HS2 Is the space safe and clear enough to work in?

HS3 Are the children aware of others in the class when they are moving and working?

HS4 Have all the children warmed up and cooled down properly?

Unit descriptor – Athletic activities (2)

Section 1: Acquiring and developing skills

Objectives – Children should learn:

- to consolidate and improve the quality, range and consistency of the techniques they use for particular activities

Table 1.6 Activities

1.1 Ask the children to run for short distances and times, and for longer distances and times. Encourage them to keep a steady pace. They could work in teams or on their own.

1.2 Ask the children to practise the five basic jumps, e.g. one foot to same foot (hop), one foot to other foot (step), one foot to two feet, two feet to two feet, two feet to one foot, as single jumps and then in simple combinations. Teach them to combine the basic jump actions and to form simple jump combinations.

Table 1.6 Activities (cont.)

1.3 Ask them to show different ways of throwing a range of equipment. Teach them to throw using slinging, pushing and pulling actions.

Outcomes

1.4 Run consistently and smoothly at different speeds.

1.5 Demonstrate different combinations of jumps, showing control, coordination and consistency.

1.6 Throw a range of implements into a target area with consistency and accuracy.

Section 2: Selecting and applying skills, tactics and compositional ideas
Objectives – Children should learn:

- to develop their ability to choose and use simple tactics and strategies in different situations

Table 1.7 Activities

2.1 Help the children to see that they are better at running at a high speed for short times and distances than for longer ones. Teach them how to pace their effort over different distances.

2.2 Help the children to see that they can throw equipment further using some methods than others. Teach them to choose the best method for the equipment they are given.

2.3 Help the children to see that different types of jump are better for getting height or distance. Teach them how to choose the best method and how to combine jumps. Ask the children to run their own athletic events and simple competitions. Show them how to judge, measure and record athletic activity. Help them to make the competitions fair.

Table 1.7 Outcomes
2.4 Recognise that there are different styles of running, jumping and throwing, and that they need to choose the best for a particular challenge and type of equipment.
2.5 Pace their effort well in different types of event so that they can keep going steadily and maintain the quality of their action.

Section 3: Knowledge and understanding of fitness and health

Objectives – Children should learn:

- to know, measure and describe the short-term effects of exercise on the body
- to describe how the body reacts to different types of activity

Table 1.8 Activities
3.1 Help the children to describe what their bodies feel like after an event. Teach them how to feel and count their heartbeat. Help them to recognise how different activities make them more or less tired.
3.2 Show the children how to record the differences in their body after different types of challenge.
3.3 Teach them stretching and other safe warm-up activities.
Outcomes
3.4 Identify and record when their body is cool, warm and hot.
3.5 Recognise and record that their body works differently in different types of challenge and event.
3.6 Carry out stretching and warm-up activities safely.

Section 4: Evaluating and improving performance
Objectives – Children should learn:

- to describe and evaluate the effectiveness of performances, and recognise aspects of performances that need improving

---

Table 1.9 Activities

4.1 Teach the children what to look at when watching someone perform, e.g. jumping or throwing action used, position of the feet in throw or jump, type of arm swing in running, length of stride used, evenness of the pace in running.

4.2 Listen to the way they describe their own and others' running, jumping and throwing actions. Help them to suggest how an action could be improved.

Outcomes

4.3 Watch and describe specific aspects of running, jumping and throwing styles.

4.4 Suggest, with guidance, a target for improving distance or height.

Key points; Health and safety

Table 1.10 Key points

KP1 In every lesson, most of the children's learning should take place through physical activity relating to the core tasks.

KP2 Most lessons should start with short warm-up activities that help the children remember what they did in the last lesson and prepare them for what they will learn next. Most lessons should end with cool-down activities.

KP3 Give the children opportunities to practise, repeat and refine the skills they learn. Vary activities so that the children don't get too tired in any one event or challenge. Organise a range of competitions for individuals and groups, e.g. the combined distance thrown in an event by a small group.

KP4 The children should set their own targets for performance. They could design a spreadsheet for recording and interpreting their results, and could also use the spreadsheet for organising competitions. Give them the opportunity to measure and record throwing and jumping activities.

Table 1.10 Key points (cont.)

KP5 Make sure the children have an opportunity to see good-quality performances by their peers and others. Encourage them to look at how movements start and finish.

KP6 Give the children specific guidance on the skills they need to use and how to use them correctly, as well as general feedback and praise. Give them opportunities to talk about what they are doing and to comment on their own and others' performances.

KP7 A CD-ROM could be used to show the human body in action, focusing in particular on muscles. This could also be linked to Unit 4A 'Moving and Growing', in the science scheme of work.

Health and safety

HS1 Do the children's clothing and footwear help their learning and keep them safe?

HS2 Are the children aware of others in the class when they are moving and working?

HS3 Is the space safe and clear enough to work in?

HS4 Have all the children warmed up and cooled down properly?

CHAPTER TWO
Child development

2

Objectives

After completing this chapter the reader should be able to:

- Explain the nature versus nurture debate.
- List and describe the various stages of child development.
- Discuss the common physiological differences between children and adults.
- List the types of bone found in the human body.
- Explain the functions of types of bone.
- Describe how bone growth occurs throughout childhood.
- Describe common childhood injuries related to bone growth.
- Identify types of muscle and describe the composition of skeletal muscle.
- List and describe different types of skeletal muscle fibre.
- Discuss fat storage throughout childhood.
- Discuss methods of measuring fat percentage, in particular BMI and the advantages and disadvantages of this method.
- Discuss the cardiovascular differences between children and adults.
- Explain how cardiovascular endurance is measured and the units used.
- List and describe the role of hormones in the endocrine system.
- Discuss the effects of training on hormone levels.
- List and describe the different components associated with psychological development.

Introduction

When talking about the growth and development of children, there is an age-old debate known as 'nature versus nurture'. In simple terms this debate considers how children are influenced both genetically (nature) by their parents and by the environment (nurture) in which they grow up: in other words, how genetics, exercise, lifestyle and nutrition can all play an important role in the development of children. However, most of the knowledge relating to the response of the human body is based on studies with adults as it is often considered unethical to carry out studies on young children. Before discussing the development of children, however, it is useful to understand some of the terms that are often used when referring to children at different stages in their lives. Table 2.1 gives a description of the various stages that will be used throughout this book.

Table 2.1 Descriptions of common terms

Stage of development	Description
Infancy	This stage of development normally refers to the first year of life
Childhood	From age 1 up to puberty
Puberty	When the development of secondary sex characteristics and the capability of sexual reproduction occurs prior to adolescence
Adolescence	From puberty to the completion of growth and development (adulthood)

The development of the human being can be broadly categorised into two areas: physiological (to do with the body) and psychological (to do with the mind). For the purpose of this book, physiological development will cover areas such as skeletal, muscular, fat, cardiovascular, hormonal and motor skill development, whereas psychological development will mainly cover the area of learning theories. Before dealing with the physiological development of children it would be useful to have a quick look at the main physiological differences between children and adults, which will then be expanded on in the following chapters. Table 2.2 shows just some of the physiological differences between children and adults.

Skeletal development

The material we call bone is what is known as 'calcified connective tissue' and is the hardest tissue in the body, which gives it strength (but when it is fully developed it is also quite light). In the adult skeleton there are approximately 206 bones (sometimes some of the bones fuse together as in the coccyx). An adult has more bones than a child: this is because bone starts out as a substance called 'cartilage', and it takes time to complete the process of turning into bone, which is called 'bone maturation' or 'ossification' ('ossi' means 'bone' and 'fication' means 'making').

Types of bone

There are several different types (or classifications as they are normally termed) of bone in the human body, as can be seen in fig. 2.1, and many bones of each of the different

Table 2.2 Main physiological differences between children and adults

Physiological effect	How children differ from adults
VO_2max (see page 37)	Lower but increases from about age 6 years up to adolescence
Stroke volume (see page 36)	Lower at a given intensity
Cardiac output (see page 36)	Lower at a given intensity
Max heart rate	Higher
Respiratory rate	Higher
Running economy	Lower
Thermal regulation	Less efficient

types. The types of bone are simply named based on their appearance and shape: long, short, flat, irregular and sesamoid. It may seem strange, but bones of the same type can look very different even though they have the same general characteristics.

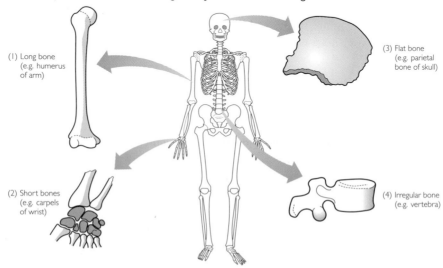

(1) Long bone (e.g. humerus of arm)

(2) Short bones (e.g. carpels of wrist)

(3) Flat bone (e.g. parietal bone of skull)

(4) Irregular bone (e.g. vertebra)

Fig. 2.1 Types of bone in the skeleton

The different types of bone tend to have different general functions. In simple terms, the long bones in the limbs (arms and legs) are the ones that grow to give us our height and also help us to move, whereas flat bones are the ones that tend to be used for protection purposes and for the attachment of large tendons (a tendon is tissue that connects the muscle to the bone). Table 2.3 gives a more detailed explanation of the functions of the different types of bone. Try the task in table 2.4 to test your knowledge of bones.

Table 2.3 Functions of types of bone		
Bone Type	**Function**	**Example**
Long	These bones comprise a shaft with two extremities. The shaft is known as the diaphysis and the extremities are known as the epiphyses. Just before each epiphysis is a region known as the growth plate or epiphyseal cartilage. This is the point in the bone at which growth occurs and when growth finally stops in adulthood the epiphyseal cartilage becomes fully developed bone. Fatty yellow bone marrow can be found within the central part of the long bone known as the medullary canal. Long bones act as levers to provide locomotion for the body as they have muscles that are attached to them that can pull and create movement. The femur and humerus are examples of long bones.	These bones are found mainly in the limbs.
Short	Short bones are designed mainly for lightness and strength. They are usually cube-shaped and are mainly spongy (cancellous) bone with a thin compact outer layer.	Short bones can be found in the wrist (carpals) and ankles (tarsals).
Flat	These are spongy (cancellous) bones sandwiched between two compact layers either giving protection as in the skull or providing a large area for muscle attachment as in the pelvis.	Pelvis, skull, scapula.
Irregular	This type of bone usually has bony projections that are there for the purpose of muscle attachment.	The vertebrae (bones of the spine).
Sesamoid	These are seed-like bones, normally pea size, that are developed within the tendon of a muscle.	Patella.

TRY THIS!
Identify a location in the body for each bone.

Femur
Tibia
Ulna
Radius
Fibula
Humerus
Tarsals
Metatarsals
Carpals
Metacarpals
Scapula
Clavicle
Patella

Growth of bones

When we go through our growth development it is the long bones in our bodies that grow in length, at the region known as the 'epiphyseal' or 'growth plate'. This region is an area of cartilage near to the end of a long bone (see fig. 2.2). If you were to look at the ends of a long bone you would see that they were covered in a hard, shiny substance. This substance is known as 'articular cartilage', which is a very tough substance that helps to protect the ends of the bone. This is essential because it is the ends of bones that come together to form a joint where there will be movement and, as a result, friction would normally occur as the ends of the bone could actually rub against each other. Excessive exercise can cause this cartilage to wear down, which eventually leads to a condition known as 'arthritis'.

Bones do not grow at a steady rate throughout life. The fastest rate of growth of bone is within the first two years of life, when a child can reach up to half of their full-grown height. Generally speaking, bone growth can continue until the early twenties at

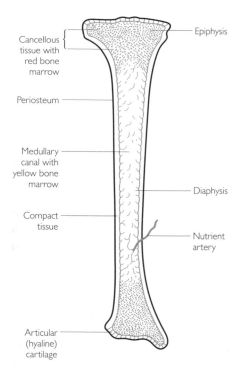

Cancellous
tissue with
red bone
marrow

Epiphysis

Periosteum

Medullary
canal with
yellow bone
marrow

Diaphysis

Compact
tissue

Nutrient
artery

Articular
(hyaline)
cartilage

Fig. 2.2 A typical long bone

an average rate of about two inches a year but is usually different for boys and girls. Girls generally mature physiologically about 2–2.5 years earlier than boys do. Growth spurts (a period when growth appears to be quicker) tend to occur at different times in life for boys and girls. For girls the main growth spurt typically occurs between the ages of 10 and 13 years. For boys, growth spurts typically occur around 12–14 years of age. As bones are still growing at this age, this often means that children are more susceptible to certain injuries as they don't have the bone strength to cope with sustained high-impact activities that they may do.

In relation to bone growth during childhood, many nutrients are required in the diet, such as calcium, vitamin C and phosphorus. As well as dietary factors affecting bone growth, hormones can also affect it at different times in life. Growth hormone and testosterone are just two of the hormones that can affect the rate of growth, particularly around puberty. Once the bones in the body stop growing, the growth plate area (which is cartilage) is then replaced by bone.

Common childhood injuries
It is known that activity can have a positive effect on bone growth but the exact amount, type and process are not completely understood. Generally, resistance and impact-type

exercises, which put force on the bone, are thought to stimulate bone growth. Care must be taken, however, as it is also known that there are several injuries that are associated with excessive activity in children, such as chondromalacia patella, Osgood-Schlatter disease, Sever's disease and growth plate injuries.

- Chondromalacia patella: The female hips are generally wider than male hips. Wide hips result in the femur (the upper leg bone) being placed at a greater inward angle than in males. This can cause injury (also known as 'runner's knee') that occurs when the patella does not run smoothly in the groove at the end of the femur. In this situation the cartilage on the back of the patella can wear away causing pain.

- Osgood-Schlatter disease: This is the name of a common condition in which the patella (knee cap) tendon pulls away from its attachment point just below the knee (the tibial tuberosity). It is usually due to excessive impact over a period of time, which eventually results in a build-up of scar tissue and subsequently causes pain.

- Sever's disease: When the Achilles tendon (this is the tendon at the back of the lower leg) repetitively pulls on its attachment point at the heel, it can also cause pain just like the patella tendon. The Achilles tendon was actually named after the Greek hero Achilles in the Trojan War. It was thought that his only weak point was his heel and so to this day we refer to someone's weak point as their Achilles heel.

- Growth plate injuries: As mentioned earlier in this chapter, bone growth occurs near the ends of long bones (epiphyseal or growth plate) so that the bone grows in length. Excessive loads at the area of the growth plate can sometimes affect bone growth.

Throughout this chapter we have taken a selection of some of the questions from the National Curriculum for PE that children are expected to be able to answer at various key stages in their development. This might help the coach relate to children when delivering activity sessions. Table 2.4 shows some of the questions at key stages 1 and 2 that are related to the skeleton.

Table 2.4 Key stage questions for the skeleton

Key stage questions	Key Stage
Are bones hard or soft?	1
Are bones strong or weak?	1
Can you name any bones?	2
How may you get hurt?	1
What do bones protect?	1
Name a bone and what it protects.	2
What joins onto bones to help us move?	2
What types of movement can we do?	1

Muscular development

When discussing the development of muscle tissue within the body, it is useful to have a general understanding of the make-up (composition as it is known) and roles of the different types of fibre relating to what we know as 'skeletal muscle'.

Types of muscle

There are actually three types of muscle tissue that can be found in the human body:

- Cardiac muscle: The heart muscle
- Smooth muscle: A squeezing-action (peristaltic) muscle, such as in the digestive system
- Skeletal muscle: A movement muscle mainly attached to bones

Each type of muscle within the body develops throughout childhood. For instance, the heart becomes larger and stronger in order to pump a greater volume of blood around a larger body. Smooth muscle in the digestive system and other places such as the arteries also develops its contraction ability in order to squeeze contents such as food and blood. However, we will focus on skeletal muscles for the purpose of this book.

SKELETAL MUSCLE

Muscles are made up of individual muscle fibres (made up of proteins), which run the entire length of the muscle. These fibres are called 'myofibrils', as can be seen in figure 2.3.

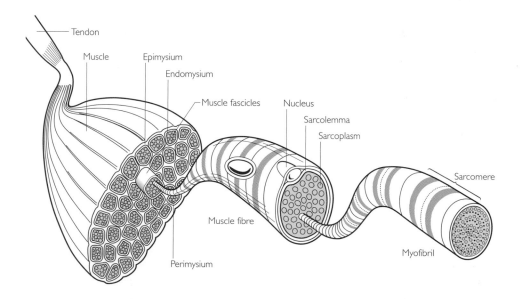

Fig. 2.3 A typical skeletal muscle structure

In some muscles there might be relatively few fibres, such as in muscles of the eye in which there are only tens of fibres. In some of the bigger muscles in the body there may be thousands of fibres. For instance, there can be up to 400,000 fibres in the biceps muscle, which is in the front of the arm. Each muscle fibre is surrounded by a sheath of fibrous tissue membrane, or fascia (meaning bandage), called the 'endomysium' ('endo' meaning 'within'). This is similar to a sausage wrapped in a skin. Muscle fibres are then grouped together in a bundle (fascicle) and surrounded by another sheath called the 'perimysium' ('peri' meaning 'around'). Finally, another sheath called the 'epimysium' ('epi' meaning 'upon') surrounds the entire muscle. At each end of the muscle the three types of sheath taper off and converge together to form an attachment to the bone. The attachment point of muscle to bone is called a tendon and when muscle contracts it pulls on the tendon, which in turn pulls on the bone and causes movement.

Skeletal muscles are known as 'voluntary'. This is because we have to think about movement to actually do it as opposed to movement being automatic (except in the case of a reflex). In terms of muscle composition, if we were able to look at a typical skeletal muscle under a microscope, we would see that it is striated (striped) in appearance. About 40–46% of body weight between the ages of 5 and 29 years is made up of muscle tissue. The largest muscle in the body is the gluteus maximus, which is the main part of the buttock. The strongest muscle is usually considered to be the quadriceps (front of the thigh) even though the jaw can create a greater force. The longest muscle in the body is the sartorius running from the iliac spine in the pelvis to the medial aspect of the tibia (top of the shin). Try the task in table 2.6 to test your muscle knowledge.

TRY THIS!
Identify a location in the body for each muscle.

Triceps
Biceps
Pectoral
Trapezius
Latissimus dorsi
Deltoid
Quadriceps
Hamstring

Calf
Tibialis anterior
Abductor
Adductor
Hip flexor

Fibre types

All muscle fibres are not exactly the same, as they have different roles within the body. There are many different types of skeletal muscle fibre but they are commonly split into two groups: fast- and slow-twitch. Slow-twitch fibres are also called Type I fibres and fast-twitch fibres are further split into Type IIa and Type IIb fibres. The differences in the fibres can be seen in table 2.5.

Human beings have different percentages of all three fibre types, depending on their genetics. It is possible to change the way fibres behave but only by a small amount; therefore we are what we were born with and training can have only a small, though sometimes crucial, effect. As with skeletal growth, the muscles in the body also grow at irregular rates. It is thought that the number of muscle fibres is genetically determined and that growth of muscle is due to enlargement of the fibres in the muscles and not to splitting or increasing the number of fibres.

Table 2.5 Common characteristics of muscle fibres

	Type I	Type IIa	Type IIb
Contraction time	Slow	Fast	Very fast
Resistance to fatigue	High	Intermediate	Low
Activity used for	Aerobic	Longer-term anaerobic	Short-term anaerobic
Force production	Low	High	Very high
Colour	Reddish	Whitish	Whitish
Blood supply	Very good	Not as good	Not so good
Main fuel	Fat	Carbohydrate	Carbohydrate

Definition

The word 'genetic' comes from the Greek word 'genesis' meaning 'birth' and was first used in the early 1900s. The word 'genes' is used to describe the characteristic building blocks of life inherited from our parents. We have many thousands of genes, which determine many different physical characteristics such as hair and eye colour.

The enlargement of muscles (known as 'hypertrophy') makes them thicker, but muscle fibres can also get longer. At puberty, boys tend to have a faster rate of muscle growth than girls due to increased levels of testosterone, which helps to build muscles. With certain types of training and genetics, boys' muscle mass can peak at about 50% of body weight around the ages of 18 to 25 years, whereas girls' muscle mass peaks at about 40% of body weight around the ages of 16 to 20 years. Table 2.6 shows some of the questions at key stages 1 and 2 that are related to the muscles.

Table 2.6 Key stage questions for muscles

Key stage questions	Key Stage
Are muscles inside or outside your body?	1
What do muscles do?	1
Can you name any muscles?	2

Fat development

Before we look at the storage of fat in the body we need to distinguish between what we call 'fat mass' and 'fat-free mass'. In simple terms, fat mass is the weight of all the fat that is stored in the body and fat-free mass is the weight of everything else that is not fat, such as bone, cartilage, muscle and blood.

Fat storage

The storage of fat starts as early as birth and continues throughout life. The human body needs a certain amount of fat, which is either used in many processes in the body or stored in fat cells around the body. The main fat storage sites are around the internal organs and underneath the skin (this is known as 'subcutaneous tissue'). Obviously, the storage of too much fat is a problem as this can lead to obesity, which is associated with many health problems. Fat storage is not just dependent on exercise and diet but also has a genetic link. In simple terms, the amount of fat in the body can influence both athletic performance and general health and is particularly significant in sports that have weight categories.

Measuring body fat

There are many different ways of estimating the amount of fat a person has, such as underwater weighing, infra-red, bio-electrical and skinfold calliper, but these methods are not often used with children, as they are considered 'invasive'. One of the most common methods used is body mass index (BMI), which is not as accurate as some of the other methods but is regarded as 'non-invasive'. All the tester has to do is measure the height and weight of the child and calculate a BMI number or score using the formula:

$$BMI = \frac{Weight\ (kg)}{Height^2\ (m^2)}$$

For adults this score is then given a BMI rating or classification using the scale proposed by ACSM shown in table 2.7.

The classification for children is different, however, because of the vast differences within the age ranges. For this reason, age-related scales are used in which the BMI score is rated on the basis of the age of the child being tested, which then gives a classification (overweight, obese etc.) for that particular child.

Table 2.7 BMI classifications for adults

BMI classification	BMI score
Acceptable	20–24.9
Overweight	25–29.9
Obese	30+
Class I obese	30–34.9
Class II obese	35–39.9
Class III obese	40+

Fat percentage

Many people do not like using BMI as a method of classifying obesity as it does not really take into account muscle tissue in the body. For this reason, an overall percentage measurement of fat in the body is preferred. As mentioned earlier, the skinfold calliper method is a simple and cheap way of measuring fat percentage but this is not recommended for use with children: a method such as bioelectrical impedance (this is an electrical device attached to the hand and foot) would be considered a better option. Putting children into categories corresponding to fat percentage is a delicate issue and the guidelines are not readily available. However, some guidelines relating to the age range of 7–18 years are shown in figure 2.4, adapted from work by Cole in 1995.

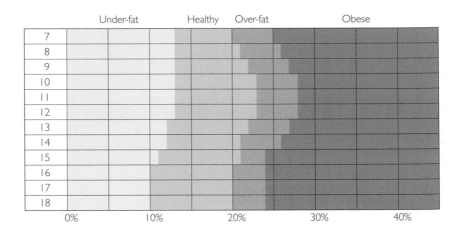

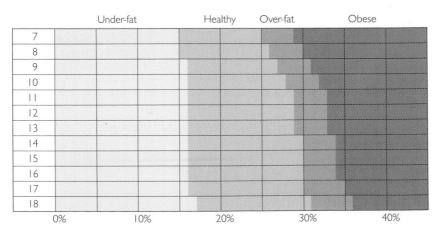

Fig. 2.4 Body fat ranges for children aged 7–18 years (a) Male 7–18 years (b) Female 7–18 years (adapted from Cole, 1995)

It is interesting to note that, with the guideline ranges for males, there appears to be a period leading up to puberty when the level of body fat can go higher before individuals are classed as being over-fat, followed by a period when the level decreases. For females, however, the situation is different as the level at which individuals are classed as being over-fat seems to increase steadily with age (with a couple of periods where it remains steady). It does need to be stressed at this point, though, that the issue of overweight, and indeed underweight, is a very delicate one and if coaches suspect there is a possible issue with a particular child, they should in most cases seek further professional guidance as any misdiagnosis in this area can have serious consequences.

Statistics

Even though the statistics for overweight and obese people are ever increasing and we are becoming a larger nation, a general rule-of-thumb for body fat amounts during childhood development (measured in percentage terms) is as follows:

- At birth: Both boys and girls have around 10–12% body fat
- Pre-puberty: Both boys and girls have around 16–18% body fat
- Post-puberty: Girls have around 25% body fat due to female hormones causing extra fat to be stored
- Post-puberty: Boys have about 12–14% body fat

As well as being overweight, being underweight can also be a problem for children (in both males and females). A body fat percentage of less than 12% for females is generally considered to be unhealthy for many reasons. Therefore, a coach should always be aware of this if working with a female who appears to be very lean. The problem with this is that the coach would need to be directly involved in the measurement of body fat; however, there are always errors involved in this kind of measurement, depending on the technique used and especially for low levels of body fat. For this reason, the coach should always use their professional judgement regarding the child by first considering speaking to the parents and then recommending that further advice be sought from a suitably qualified person.

Did you know ?

The only direct method of measuring body fat is to dissect dead bodies.

Cardiovascular development

Before exploring this particular topic we need to clarify what is meant by 'cardiovascular'. The term 'cardiovascular' simply relates to the heart and all the vessels associated with it (arteries, veins and capillaries).

Children versus adults

In relation to the ability of the heart and its vessels, there are many differences between children and adults. For instance, the stroke volume (SV) and cardiac output (CO) are lower in children than in adults at any given level of activity. In other words, children cannot pump the same amount of blood around the body in the same time period as adults, because they have smaller heart chambers and lower blood volume than adults.

Definition
- 'Stroke volume' is the volume of blood pumped out of the heart in one contraction.
- 'Cardiac output' is the total volume of blood pumped out of the heart in one minute.

Heart rate also tends to be higher in children than in adults. Heart rate is simply a term for how many times the heart beats in a given time period, usually one minute. During the same level of exercise, a child would need to work harder than an adult, as a child can only supply a fraction of the oxygen requirements of the muscles involved in comparison to adults (it is this supply of oxygen to the muscle that helps it to do work). This can be seen in figure 2.5, which shows that an adult heart does not have to beat as fast for the same level of exercise, as it is bigger and can supply more oxygen with each beat. That is why older children do not appear to be working as hard as the younger children during activities in which they are all participating (assuming the fitness levels are all reasonably equal). It is important for the coach to understand that younger children, therefore, can only sustain high levels of exercise or activity for short periods of time, although this will develop as they get older and fitter.

Did you know
An adult heart pumps enough blood every day to fill about 30 baths.

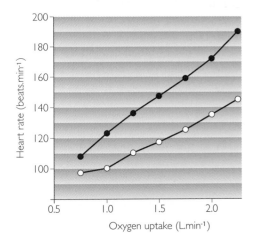

Fig. 2.5 Typical heart rates for a boy and a man for different levels of exercise

Measuring cardiovascular fitness

The amount or volume of oxygen (VO_2) that can be supplied to the muscles in the body during exercise is normally used as an indication of fitness levels. As can be seen in figure 2.6, if the intensity of the exercise is increased gradually (running speed for example), the volume of oxygen needed will also increase gradually. At a certain point, depending on the individual, the amount of oxygen that can be supplied to the muscles will reach a maximum – this measurement is called VO_2max.

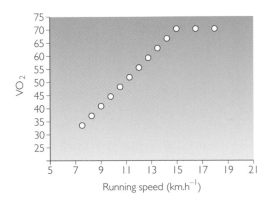

Fig. 2.6 Relationship between exercise intensity and volume of oxygen (VO_2)

It makes sense, therefore, that the more oxygen that an individual can get to their muscles to provide energy, the fitter they will be. This measurement of fitness is usually greater in boys than in girls and peaks at different ages: VO_2max tends to reach its peak around the age of 17 to 21 years in males and decreases with age, whereas it has been shown to reach its peak around the age of 12 to 15 years in females, though the general decrease after the age of 15 years may be due to the tendency for females to reduce their amount of regular physical activity.

Did you know
If all the blood vessels in the body were joined end to end they could wrap four times round the earth!

Even though the measurement of VO_2max is considered to be neither ethical nor useful for younger children, it is something that tends to be done on a regular basis, probably without the testers involved even knowing that they are doing it. I am sure you are familiar with the 'bleep test', or the 'multi-stage fitness test' as it is better known. This test is commonly performed on a regular basis in schools throughout the UK, even for children as young as 10 years of age. It is actually classed as a maximal test in that participants are asked to run for as long as they possibly can until they fatigue. In many cases, children who participate will push themselves to the limit and hence reach maximum heart rate levels. The idea is that each participant runs backwards and forwards on a 20-metre course and runs faster and faster in order to keep up with a 'bleep' sound, which speeds up at higher and higher levels. Once the participant can no longer keep up, they drop out at a particular level. That level can then be converted to a VO_2max score by using a conversion table, which is split only into male and female categories and not into age ranges. I have had experience of my own son coming home with the taste of iron (from blood) in his mouth after completely exhausting himself during a bleep test.

Did you know
The left lung is smaller than the right one so that there is space for the heart.

It is important, therefore, that coaches de-emphasise the importance of measurements such as VO$_2$max and concentrate on other components of fitness and performance of skills and technique during the early years and then on cardiovascular fitness at later stages of childhood. Table 2.8 shows some of the questions at key stages 1 and 2 that are related to cardiovascular development.

Table 2.8 Key stage questions for cardiovascular development

Key stage questions	Key Stage
What can you feel beating in your chest?	1
How can we get air into our bodies?	**1 and 2**
What carries the energy around our bodies?	2
How may you get hurt?	1
What do bones protect?	1
Name a bone and what it protects.	2
What joins onto bones to help us move?	2
What types of movement can we do?	1

Hormonal development

During childhood the production and levels of molecules known as 'hormones' increase in the body. The physiological system that is responsible for the production and release of hormones is known as the 'endocrine system'.

Definition

The word 'hormone' is taken from the Greek word meaning 'impetus' or 'excitement' and is simply a chemical messenger in the body.

The endocrine system

The endocrine system is simply a messenger system for the body that is capable of sending messages by using hormones secreted by glands, organs or specialised tissues. This is normally done in conjunction with the nervous system whereby if the homeostasis[1] of the body is disturbed, it is recognised by the nervous system (remember the sensory

[1] Taken from the Greek word homoios meaning similar, this refers to the body keeping the internal systems stable regardless of the external environment.

receptors are responsible for this), which in turn stimulates specific glands in the body to release hormones that function in order to return the body to homeostasis. Most hormones are circulated via the bloodstream and therefore this system can be quite slow, compared to the nervous system in which the messages sent are very fast. The main endocrine glands in the body include the pineal, pituitary, thyroid, parathyroid and adrenal glands. There are other tissues that secrete hormones, such as the hypothalamus, pancreas, thymus, ovaries, testes, kidneys and stomach, but are not referred to as endocrine glands. Figure 2.7 gives an overview of the roles of the main hormones in the body.

Pituitary	Produces mainly trophic hormones (i.e. hormones that stimulate other glands) and growth hormone.
Pineal	Releases melatonin to promote sleep.
Thyroid	Controls metabolism.
Parathyroid	Controls metabolism. Produces hormones that control bone growth by regulating calcium levels in the body.
Adrenal	Produce adrenalin, cortisol and noradrenaline which are responsible for the increase in nutrient breakdown.
Pancreas	Responsible for the release of insulin into the bloodstream in order to reduce blood sugar levels.
Testes and ovaries	Produce sex hormones such as testosterone and oestrogen to regulate reproductive function.

Fig. 2.7 Main hormones and their roles

One of the main hormones that is found in females is known as 'oestrogen'. This particular hormone is associated with mood changes and feelings of self-consciousness. Oestrogen is also known to stimulate bone growth and fat deposits. The hormonal changes that occur around the age of puberty can also affect body composition in terms of the amount of fat that is stored. At birth and up to puberty, both boys and girls have a similar body fat percentage but, post-puberty, girls' levels increase to around 25% (much higher than in boys) due to high oestrogen levels, which cause the hips to widen and extra fat to be stored in the same area. One of the main hormones found in males (and some females) is 'testosterone', which is known to be responsible for stimulating bone and muscle growth but can also result in competitiveness and aggression (as does growth hormone (GH)).

Did you know

The hips in females widen to allow for childbirth later in life!

Response to training

Even though it is difficult to study the response of the endocrine system (and the asso-ciated hormones) to training, some research studies have shown that there is a hormonal adaptation in relation to the intensity and duration when doing resistance-type training. As can be seen in figure 2.7, the endocrine system can play a vital role in the body by regulating functions such as metabolism and growth and can also be instrumental in affecting the mood state of an individual. The endocrine system can also play a major role in muscle adaptations to exercise (in particular resistance training). Depending on the type of training and the individual, resistance training can cause increased levels of anabolic (building up) hormones such as testosterone and GH and decreased levels of catabolic (breaking down) hormones such as cortisol. However, it has been shown that strength training can increase testosterone levels in both young and older males, but not always in females.

Generally speaking, it seems that the greater the volume of resistance training that is done (using medium loads and relatively short recovery periods), the greater the increase in production of testosterone (with Olympic lifts, squats and dead lifts producing the greatest increases). Interestingly, resistance training using heavy loads and longer recovery periods (1–3 repetition maximum (RM) and 5–8 min recovery) tends to result in smaller increases in testosterone than those observed from training using medium loads. Maybe it is this effect that can explain why those individuals training to increase muscle mass are normally advised to use moderate loads, several sets and a short recovery, rather than purely maximal strength training. Coaches must be wary, therefore, not to embark on a programme of muscle-building resistance training exercises for children especially around the age of puberty, since hormones in the body are already at peak levels as can easily be detected by the common mood swings that will occur as a result.

Psychological development

There are many components that could contribute to the psychological development of the child but, for the purpose of this book, figure 2.8 shows the areas that will be consid-ered. Each area will only be covered briefly as coaches should be aware that there is a great deal of information relating to each one. Therefore further study should be considered if the coach has an interest in any particular area.

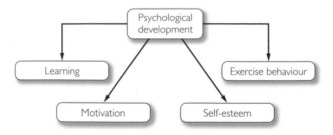

Fig. 2.8 Components contributing to psychological development

Learning

Like all adaptations that occur in the body, there are many theories relating to how we as human beings learn. These theories can generally be classified into two main groups that are known as 'cognitive theories' or 'behaviourist theories'.

Definition

The word 'cognitive' derives from the Latin tem 'cognoscere' meaning 'to know' and is the scientific term used for thinking or the process of thinking.
Behaviourist theories are more to do with the reaction to a stimulus which takes away the need for thinking.

The scientist Edward Lee Thorndike (1874–1949) is often associated with the development of the behaviourist theory of learning. In general terms, he stated that learning occurs by trial and error and there is an association between the stimulus and the response. This led to a simplistic view that responses resulting in a positive or satisfying experience are more likely to be repeated, whereas responses resulting in a negative or annoying experience are less likely to be repeated. This thinking was challenged by other more recent scientists and led to the development of new behaviourist theories that are used today. Some of the behaviourist theories include classical conditioning (stimulus–response), operant conditioning (stimulus not always needed) and drive reduction.

- Classical conditioning: A scientist called Ivan Pavlov (1849–1936) discovered that if he rang a bell when feeding dogs, they were eventually conditioned to salivate (drool) at the sound of the bell (even if no food followed). This demonstrated that a response (the drooling) can be associated with a specific stimulus (the bell ringing) and was given the name 'classical conditioning', on which much research has been conducted by the scientist John Watson. This type of conditioning is often used in sporting situations when the coach wants to change the response of a performer in a certain situation, such as for controlling anxiety when taking a penalty kick. For instance, sportspeople often use phrases such as 'breathe easy', which can help to induce muscular relaxation when the sportsperson is in an anxious state.

- Operant conditioning: Another scientist, B.F. Skinner (1903–1990), demonstrated that behaviour can occur without an obvious stimulus. He did this by putting a food dispenser with a lever above a cage with a rat in it. Every time the rat pushed the lever, food would drop out. This demonstrated that you don't necessarily require a stimulus, but can condition using reward and punishment – this was called 'operant conditioning'.
- Drive reduction: This particular theory was first put forward by C. L. Hull in 1943. He stated that learning is due to the development of habits and therefore, as a problem arises in sport that requires a response, the performer is stimulated to solve the problem – in other words, driven to learn. It is this drive to learn that encourages the performer to start practising the skill. As the performance gets better (more consistent) because of the practice, the drive to learn is reduced.

In contrast and in challenge to the behaviourist theories, a scientist called Albert Bandura, born in 1925, put forward ideas on cognitive theories, which place more emphasis on the thought process of the individual than on the reaction to a stimulus. Over the years, two main cognitive theories have emerged: social cognitive theory and situated learning theory.

- Social cognitive theory: Observational learning is considered to be a form of cognitive learning and is based on children copying the actions of others; it has been shown that children are more likely to copy models similar to themselves or models they had seen being rewarded for their actions (this is known as 'vicarious learning'). Bandura said that learning could also take place by 'doing', which is known as 'enactive learning'.
- Situated learning theory: Scientists called Lave and Wenger have put forward the notion that learning is social and takes place in a 'community of practice', which enables the learner to develop in a social setting.

Motivation

The word 'motivate' is derived from the Latin meaning 'move', which makes sense as we normally associate the result of motivation with movement of some kind. Like many psychological concepts, motivation is difficult to describe but it is generally linked to things that affect or influence our behaviour. In other words, motivation is something that can prompt a person to act in a particular way. For example, this could be something that helps someone to make lifestyle changes in order to effect weight loss or it could be something that helps another person to increase their cardiovascular fitness level (see chapter 4) in order to be competitive in sport.

There are many methods which coaches use (and sometimes they are not even aware they are using them) that are successful in motivating individuals to participate in activity and to keep coming back. On the whole, motivation is different for children than it is for adults. Adults may be highly motivated for competition reasons, or those new to exercise or activity may be motivated by factors such as weight loss. Children, on the other hand, are motivated by factors such as fun, socialising and rewards. These motivational factors may come from external sources such as a coach or a partner, or from internal factors such as the individual themselves. These types of motivation are commonly referred to as 'extrinsic' and 'intrinsic' motivation.

- Extrinsic motivation: This term is used when individuals are motivated by external rewards such as certificates, T-shirts, medals and trophies. It is no secret that children love badges, gold stars and smiley faces. External rewards can be motivational providing they are not the only reason for taking part in the activity. It is also important for adherence reasons to make sure that individuals are not over-reliant on external rewards but try to focus on internal motivational factors as well.
- Intrinsic motivation: This term is used to describe when an individual is motivated by factors such as enjoyment, fun or self-satisfaction. This type of motivation can be linked to positive feelings of self-achievement and self-esteem.

Did you know

When Muhammad Ali fought George Foreman in the 'thriller in Manila' he used several motivational techniques. One of them was to visit all the surrounding villages to drum up support before the fight. When he spoke to the villagers he got them to practise the chant 'Ali, bombaye' which meant 'Ali, kill him'. On the night of the fight over 100,000 people were to be heard chanting this phrase. This, no doubt, would have given Ali a huge lift and he went on to win the fight even though he was the massive underdog.

Self-esteem

There are many possible areas that could be considered under the heading of the psychological development of children. Even though no one area is more important than any other, we are going to take a look at one of them – a concept known as 'self-esteem'. Rather than quote an actual definition of self-esteem, it will suffice to just describe what it is. As young children develop they form an opinion or an image of themselves normally based on how others see them (not just in sporting situations but in everyday life as well). This opinion of ourselves is what we term 'self-esteem'. Even though it is considered to be a very complicated concept, it has been shown that there are many things (factors as we call them in scientific terms) that can influence an individual's perception of self-esteem. Although there are many more factors that could be considered, figure 2.9 shows an example of just some of the possibilities that have a direct influence on self-esteem.

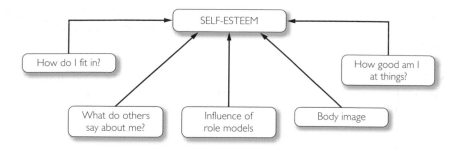

Fig. 2.9 Factors that affect self-esteem

Self-esteem in sport or activity is often linked to what happens in practice or training. For instance, if a child has a bad experience during an activity (being made to look incompetent for example), this could lead to a reduction in their self-esteem and, as a consequence, they may not want to participate in any further activity sessions. It is critical, therefore, to provide young children with a positive and encouraging environment in which they can develop and continue to participate. For this reason, coaches should always try to devise sessions that include all children (this is known as being 'inclusive') and not criticise any of them if they do not perform well at a particular skill or technique. It is usually down to the skill and experience of the coach to try to find ways to make sure that all children have some sort of success in every activity session (no matter how small) in order to give them the opportunity to feel that they fit in and that they are not being 'talked about' by other children. This approach will also help children to feel that they have been good or successful at some things, which will hopefully encourage them to come back and take part in the activities again. Finally, it is also generally thought that some sort of success, in relation to sports or activities, on a regular basis, plays a major role in building the confidence of young children, which can only positively influence their self-esteem.

Exercise behaviour

The way that children participate or not in activity or exercise is sometimes known as 'exercise behaviour'. There are many possible reasons why children would start participating in a particular activity and then why they either continue with (adhere to) that activity or just drop out of it. Children might have more than one reason to take up and maintain a particular activity and it is common for these reasons to change over a period of time. Table 2.9 lists just some of the common reasons why children might want to join in an activity and keep coming back to take part in it.

There are many theories relating to changing exercise behaviour (these are called 'behavioural change' models). However, these theories apply more to older children and adults, so coaches should just be aware of the main reasons why children would want to keep coming back and they could try to facilitate this. One of the main reasons why children adhere to exercise or activities appears to be enjoyment, or simply having fun. For many years

Table 2.9 Common reasons for children participating in and adhering to activities

Take up	Come back
Looks fun	Enjoyment
Join in with friends	Varied activities
Join in with family	Self-esteem
Play at school	Social
Don't want to be left out	Help others
Make new friends	Role model
My role model does it	I'm good at it

psychologists have known about and studied the link between having fun and arousal (this link is also known as the Yerkes-Dodson Law). This potential link makes a difference in sport and activity as it has been shown that when arousal levels in children are low, they get bored very easily. There can also be a negative situation, however: when arousal levels are high it has been shown that this can cause fear and anxiety. In other words, there appears to be an optimum arousal level (not too low and not too high) as shown in figure 2.10.

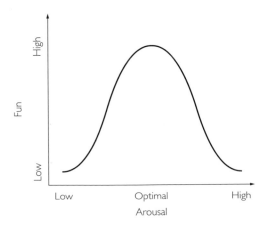

Fig. 2.10 Relationship between fun and arousal

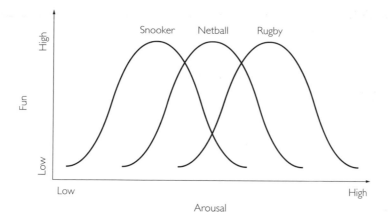

Fig. 2.11 Relationship between fun and arousal for different sports

As can be seen in figure 2.10, activities should be made fun, but coaches should be aware that too much fun might not be such a good idea, so a compromise between fun and instruction must be found. Sports psychologists often tell us that having optimal arousal levels in activities is good because children tend to focus and concentrate better on the activity when this is the case. It should be noted, however, that not all sports need high levels of arousal: there are certain sports that are usually performed better when the performer has a low level of arousal. For instance, sports such as snooker or archery would probably not be performed too well if the arousal levels of the performers were high. On the other hand, sports such as rugby or tennis would not be performed too well if the arousal levels of the performers were low. Figure 2.11 helps to depict this.

Not only do different sports often have a requirement for different levels of arousal, but all children differ in the arousal levels that suit them as individuals. Coaches need to be aware that too much fun or motivation can cause anxiety for some children. This is normally linked to the fear of failure, so it would be wise for the coach to emphasise not the winning but the taking part when trying to motivate children, which is the common approach taken throughout this book.

CHAPTER THREE
Motor skill development

Objectives

After completing this chapter the reader should be able to:

- Briefly define the term 'motor skill'.
- List and describe the different categories of motor skills.
- Define the term 'multi-skills' and list and describe the different categories.
- Discuss the development of multi-skills in relation to age.
- Identify teaching points for a range of multi-skills.
- Identify and describe different types of skill practice.
- Define the term 'skill acquisition' and related theories, in particular the three-step model of learning.
- Discuss Bayli's long-term athletic development model.

Introduction

A researcher by the name of McGill described a skill as 'a task that has a specific goal'. As he did a lot of research in the sports environment, he then went on to say that skills in sport have movement associated with them and so the term 'motor skill' was used. In other words, motor skills could also be referred to as 'movement skills'. His definition of a motor skill then became 'a skill that requires voluntary body movement to achieve the goal'. Research in the area of motor skills is vast and can often be confusing due to the large number of terms used, especially when trying to classify motor skills. Despite this, most sources agree that, even though it is difficult to classify all the different types of motor skill, they can generally be grouped into several main categories, or types.

Categories of motor skills

All motor skills fall into one of two main groups: 'gross motor skills' or 'fine motor skills'. However, there are further ways to describe motor skills by using other terms such as open, closed, internally or externally paced, discrete, serial and continuous. Table 3.1 gives a brief description of each of these possible categories.

Table 3.1 Descriptions of categories of motor skill

Category	Description	Example
Gross	Skills involving large movements in which the major muscle groups are used. The movements are not very precise.	Fundamental movement patterns such as walking, running and jumping.
Fine	Skills that involve precise movements using smaller muscle groups and generally involve high levels of hand-eye coordination.	Darts throwing, snooker and racing driving.
Open	This is where the environment is constantly changing so movements have to be continually adapted.	A pass in football under pressure from a defender.
Closed	A more predictable environment. Movements tend to follow set patterns.	A free throw in basketball, serving in tennis and a line-out in rugby.
Internally paced	Known as self-paced skills – the performer controls the speed of the skill.	These are usually closed skills – a snooker shot or a javelin throw.
Externally paced	This is where the environment or situation determines the speed of the skill. It often involves a reaction to a stimulus.	These are usually open skills – reacting to a drop shot in badminton.
Discrete	Skills which have a clear beginning and end.	A penalty kick in sports such as football and rugby.
Serial	A group of discrete skills strung together to make a more complex movement.	A triple jump or a gymnastic vault.
Continuous	Skills having no obvious beginning or end as they are repeated continuously.	Running, swimming and cycling.

It is important for the coach to remember, however, that all sports or activities are made up of a variety of different skills, and that a particular motor skill doesn't fit into just one category but can actually fall into several of them when being described. Try completing the motor skill category test in table 3.2 by placing a tick in the boxes that best describe the motor skill. The first motor skill has been done for you so you just need to complete the rest of the table.

Table 3.2 Motor skill category test

TRY THIS!
For each skill below place a tick in the box or boxes that it relates to.

	Fine	Gross	Open	Closed	Internally paced	Externally paced	Discrete	Serial	Continuous
Snooker shot	✓			✓	✓		✓		
Lineout throw									
Sprint start									
Cycle race									
Darts shot									
Free throw									
Golf putt									
Marathon run									
800m swim									

It is a useful exercise for coaches to complete the skills category test for the sport or activity that they are involved in. If they do that, they should be able to design activities for training purposes that have similar categories to those in actual game or event settings. For example, as you can see from table 3.2, snooker is a sport that requires fine-, closed-, discrete- and internal-type skills: during practice, therefore, drills that are also fine, closed, discrete and internal should be developed as they mimic the requirements of the actual sport. This can get quite complicated, however, as there are sports that incorporate many skills which can be quite different in terms of the skill classification. The coach will need to prioritise which skills to develop and concentrate on certain ones rather than trying to develop many different types of skill at the same time. It would also be advisable to try to group together skills that were in the same category for practice purposes. For instance, a weekly period of activity sessions could be made up of skills that were categorised as fine, closed, discrete and internal, whereas in the next weekly period the sessions could be made up of skills that were categorised as gross, open, continuous and external.

Definition

For the purpose of this book, the term 'multi-skills' can be thought of as the range of individual skills that are required to perform tasks such as sports or athletic events.

Multi-skills

The term 'multi-skills' is now becoming quite common in schools and sports clubs and is usually used to describe a range of motor skills that are important to learn before playing sport, as these are the component parts of what we call sport. In other words, all sports can be broken down into smaller parts, or multi-skills. There are several programmes, such as the 'BASE' programme and 'Fundamentals', that have been specifically developed as multi-skills programmes for children and are currently being adopted by many schools in the UK. It is generally agreed that introducing children as young as possible to skills is important as this provides the basis for all motor development.

It has often been demonstrated that multi-skills can develop considerably with age and especially in the first two decades of life. After the first few years of life, it is thought that all skills are then built on existing ones. It has also been demonstrated that adult skills (complex sports skills) taught too early in the child's development may create technical problems at a later stage in life. It is important, therefore, that all coaches try to introduce as wide a variety of skills as possible, to give every child the opportunity to develop these multi-skills but being mindful that they should not be too complex in the early stages.

Multi-skills menu

When working with any children, it is important to be aware of the range of multi-skills that should be taught prior to progressing to more complex and challenging ones. There are many different multi-skills that have been identified by a variety of sources over the years, so, for the purpose of this book, a range of common skills has been adapted from them, which we will call 'the multi-skills menu'. These multi-skills can be thought of as fundamental to most activities (not just sport) that children normally take part in. The multi-skills have been put into three main categories: movement skills, balance skills and manipulative skills. Table 3.3 gives a description of the skills in each category of the multi-skills menu: coaches should be aware, however, that this menu is by no means a definitive list.

Table 3.3 The multi-skills menu

Movement skills	Balance skills	Manipulative skills
Walking and jogging	Rotating the upper body	Throwing with one or both hands
Running and jumping (taking off from both feet)	Bending from the waist	Catching with one or both hands
Hopping (on both feet) and skipping	Swaying (or moving the centre of mass)	Kicking with either foot in turn
Sliding (using both feet at the front)	Squatting down	Swinging (and striking)
Galloping	Pushing and pulling with one or both hands	Bouncing with one or both hands

Development of multi-skills

The school curriculum is a useful analogy to highlight how skills should be developed. Subjects in the school curriculum are based on simple to complex progression. In mathematics, for example, numeral identification, numeral writing, numeral value identification, addition, subtraction, multiplication and division are taught in this order as each area is based on the one before it.

Taking part in sports and games activities is a similar concept. All sports are made up of individual movement, balance and manipulative skills, which all blend together to make up the complex movement patterns that are evident in all sports and games activities. As with all areas of child development, multi-skills development is individual to the child; however, there are generalisations that can be made in relation to the type of skill performed and the typical age range in which it normally occurs. For example, table 3.4 gives the general age at which certain multi-skills are usually performed.

Table 3.4 Typical multi-skills in relation to age

Age	Multi-skill
18 months	Climb up obstacles (but not back down) and also walk backwards and forwards
18 months to 2 years	Gallop
2 years	Jump up and down on the spot with both feet
2 years	Roll and kick a ball on the floor
3 years	Balance on one foot for short periods
3 years	Throw objects under-arm and also hop and skip
4 years	Balance on one foot for longer periods
4 years	Throw objects over-arm as well as under-arm
5 to 8 years	Run, hop, throw etc. with better precision

As all coaches should be providing the opportunity for children to learn these multi-skills, simple teaching points have been developed for each one to make it easier for them to coach. Using the analogy of a chef creating a dish from a variety of ingredients, if any of the fundamental or essential ingredients are missed out, the dish will be less than perfect as a result. Taking part in sports and games activities is much the same. If some of the ingredients (in this case multi-skills) are missing, it is obvious that the performance will not be so good. For this reason, it is important that all multi-skills are practised before progressing to more complex tasks such as sport.

Movement skills teaching points

Each of the movement skills (sometimes called 'locomotor skills' or 'movement concepts') can be taught using simple teaching points for ease of application within a practical environment. It is essential to use language appropriate to the level of the subject group when trying to communicate the teaching points. When giving teaching points to correct movement, use the GET correction procedure – general comment, eye contact, talk directly to the individual (*see* chapter 6). Figures 3.1 to 3.8 give a description of the various movement skills. The photos show children/adolescents from various age groups, to show how the exercises can be useful for any age.

FIG. 3.1 WALKING

- Point the feet straight ahead
- Stay relaxed and walk heel to toe and with the head up
- Swing the arms in opposition to the legs

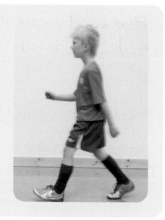

FIG. 3.2 JOGGING

- Point the feet straight ahead
- Only one foot on the ground (heel, mid-foot, ball of foot)
- Swing the arms in opposition to the legs
- Bend the elbows and relax the upper body

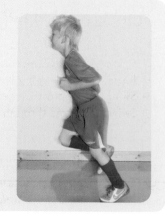

FIG. 3.3 RUNNING

- Point the feet straight ahead
- Only one foot on the ground with no heel contact
- Swing the arms in opposition to the legs
- Bend the elbows and relax the upper body

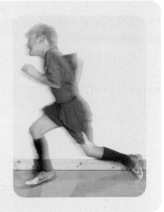

FIG. 3.4 JUMPING

- Lean forwards and swing the arms behind the body before the jump
- Take off on the toes and swing both arms forwards during the jump
- Land heels first (one or both feet) with bent knees

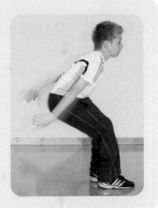

FIG. 3.5 HOPPING

- Take off and land on one foot, landing on the ball of the foot
- Keep the hopping leg slightly bent
- Swing the opposite knee through on each hop
- Swing the arms through to help drive forwards

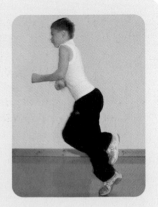

FIG. 3.6 SKIPPING

- Hop from one leg to the other
- Take off from heel to toe and land on the ball of the foot
- Bend the elbows and swing the arms in opposition to the legs

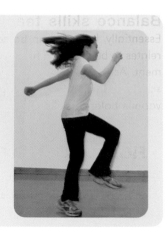

FIG. 3.7 SLIDING

- Slide on the balls of the feet
- Bend the knees and extend the arms to balance
- Lean away from the direction of motion

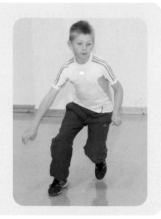

FIG. 3.8 GALLOPING

- Lean forwards slightly
- Leading leg stays forwards of the body and the back leg does not cross the front
- Heel to toe motion for the front leg and the ball of the foot for the back leg

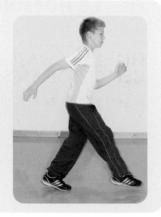

Balance skills teaching points

Essentially, balance can be categorised as either 'static' or 'dynamic'. 'Static balance' relates to balance in a fixed position, whereas 'dynamic balance' is a component of movement. As with all skills, balance or stability skills (sometimes known as 'non-locomotor' skills) can be improved through repetition. Figures 3.9 to 3.14 give a description of the various balance skills.

FiG. 3.9 ROTATING THE UPPER BODY

- Keep the feet hip-width apart
- Rotate from the thoracic spine and keep the hips still
- Maintain a neutral spine throughout

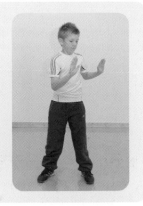

FIG. 3.10 BENDING FROM THE WAIST

- Maintain a neutral spine throughout
- Avoid excessive lean
- Encourage a comfortable range

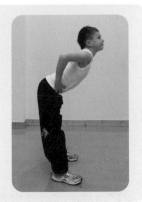

FIG. 3.11 SWAYING (SHIFTING THE CENTRE OF MASS)

- Shift the weight through the hips
- Use the arms to counterbalance
- Explore with a narrow stance then a wider one

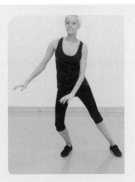

FIG. 3.12 SQUATTING DOWN

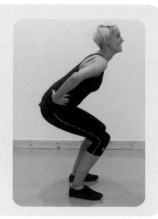

- Keep the feet hip-width apart and descend as if sitting down
- Encourage full range of motion (to the floor if possible)
- Imagine taking the ears in a straight line to the floor
- If the heels rise off the floor, encourage calf flexibility

FIG. 3.13 PUSHING

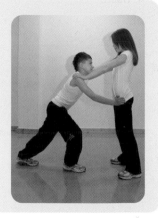

- Encourage a firm base of support to start
- Push with the whole body rather than just the arms

FIG. 3.14 PULLING

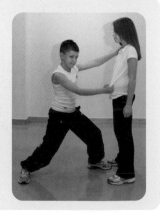

- Encourage a firm base of support to start
- Pull with the whole body rather than just the arms

Manipulative skills teaching points

Manipulation of an object with the feet, hands or other parts of the body can be one of the most challenging tasks for any person to perform, let alone a child. Hand-to-eye and foot-to-eye coordination and the ability to recover from unstable positions are among many skills that need to be mastered before effective manipulative skills can be attained. Figures 3.15 to 3.19 give a description of the various manipulative skills.

FIG. 3.15 THROWING

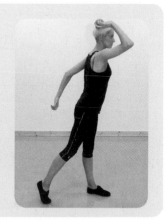

- Step into the throw with the leg in opposition to the throwing arm
- Try with and without a backswing of the arm
- Lead with the elbow (over-arm) and point the fingers towards the target
- Use a whole-body movement

FIG. 3.16 CATCHING

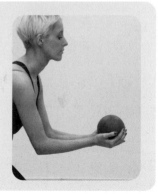

- Watch the object at all times and move towards it
- Relax the hands on impact, with the palms facing the object
- Hands flat for a high catch and pointed downwards for a low catch

FIG. 3.17 KICKING

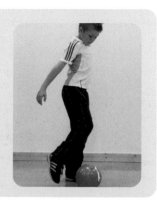

- Step into the ball when ready and bend the non-kicking leg
- Make contact with different parts of the foot and follow through
- Use a whole-body movement
- Start with a stationary ball and progress to a moving one

FIG. 3.18 SWINGING (AND STRIKING)

- Use a side orientation with the writing hand further down the bat
- Step into the swing and turn the hips
- Follow through in the direction of the target

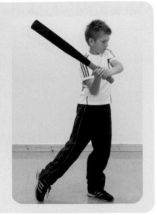

FIG. 3.19 BOUNCING

- Lean forwards slightly
- Push the ball with the finger tips – don't slap it
- Bounce at waist height and with the head up when comfortable

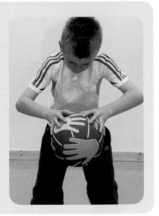

Types of practice

Regardless of the classification of the skill, it is important that all young children are given the opportunity to practise as many different skills as they possibly can. This is not as simple as it may seem, however, as there are different methods of practice that are available to the coach and the learner. The most commonly agreed classifications of methods used to practise skills are variable, fixed, massed and distributed practice. Table 3.5 gives a description of each of the types.

It is important that children should be exposed not only to all different types of skill, but also to the different types of practice in which they can use them. This is

Practice	**Description**
Variable	This refers to practising a skill in a variety of different contexts or situations and is normally used for open skills, for example practising a variety of drop shots from a half-court return in tennis.
Fixed	This is where a specific movement is practised repeatedly. This type of practice is used for skills that do not require adapting to the environment, such as closed skills. An example would be practising penalty kicks to the same corner every time.
Massed	This is where a skill is practised continuously over a period of time with few or no breaks. These sessions are often used for fixed practice skills.
Distributed	This refers to when practice is interspersed with breaks, which can be either rest or a different skill practice. This is often used with children to prevent boredom and works well.

Table 3.5 Descriptions of types of practice

because the range of sports and events favoured by children varies dramatically. As a general rule, however, variable practice (same skill but different situations) should not be used too much with those children who are new to the skills being taught, as there is much more chance of them making mistakes. If it happens that children do make mistakes, this could result in them associating the skills with a negative experience, which should be avoided as much as possible. It is also thought that massed practice (continuous practice with few or no breaks) should generally be used for older and more competitive children, as it requires a certain amount of dedication and adherence to do this type of practice as opposed to that required for distributed practice (practice with lots of breaks).

In summary, therefore, any general training programme for children of a younger age should attempt to address all types of skill but routinely swap between variable and fixed practice, while avoiding massed practice for younger children and moving from distributed to massed when they become older and more competitive.

Skill acquisition

The term 'skill acquisition' just relates to the learning of skills (in this case, motor skills). The scientific theories relating to acquiring skills usually agree that skill acquisition is slow in the early stages, followed by rapid progress. This could be due to trial and error learning, which causes the learner to constantly think about what is happening and to suddenly discover what needs to be learned by thinking about the whole process. It is interesting that some scientists recommend that skills be taught as a whole and not in parts and that the learner should practise the skill in its fullest entirety and focus on the action. This particular theory is not widely accepted by coaches, however: some think skills should be broken down and when learned, put back together (known as 'whole-part-whole'). One theory of learning that is widely taught is Schmidt's schema theory. This particular theory suggests that every time movement is produced, items of information relating to that movement are stored (a bit like a master file). This information is then grouped into four areas: conditions, body, results and feeling. These areas are described in table 3.6.

Table 3.6 Information areas of schema theory

Information area	Description
Conditions	The initial conditions relating to the movement (indoor, outdoor, sunny, cloudy, competition, practice etc.)
Body	The position of the limbs; how much force, speed etc. was used
Result	The outcome or result (was the target hit, what path did the ball take etc.)
Feeling	What the movement felt like (smooth, jerky, suddenly stopped, gradually stopped etc.)

Schmidt suggested that, by regularly practising these various movements, sets of movements (or 'schema' as he called them) are stored in the brain. These schemas are then developed and subsequently used to compare against when future movements are performed (almost like working against a model of good practice). One of the main suggestions made by Schmidt (after many years of research in this area) with regard to the type of practice used is that variable practice is more effective for skill learning than constant practice. He also suggested that the learning of a skill can be transferred from one situation to another. For example, if a hop off one foot is practised and learned, it could be used in many situations such as in the triple jump, high jump, long jump or even taking off for a lay-up basketball shot or for a header in football.

Did you know

It has been shown that academic ability is linked to fitness levels. In other words, the fitter you are, the smarter you tend to be!

Stages of learning

One of the other problems facing many coaches is how to know when a child has learned a skill so that they can progress to other or more complex skills. One of the theories of learning that can help the coach in this respect is the 'stages of learning' theory first developed by the researchers Fitts and Posner. Their theory suggests that in practice there are three distinct stages that occur when an individual is learning a new motor skill. Table 3.7 shows these stages of learning and gives a description of each.

Table 3.7 Stages of learning

Stage	Description	Example
Cognitive	The person has to consciously think about each action.	Where should my supporting leg be when kicking or how do I grip the handle for a backhand?
Associative	The person tries to detect, identify and eliminate their own errors.	I kicked the ball too high because my supporting leg was too far back.
Autonomous	The skill is performed almost as a reaction without any thought.	Wow! I just played that forehand drive without even thinking!

The stages of learning table shows that when young children are introduced to new skills they have to grasp the idea of where their limbs should be in order to do the skill (in other words, think about it!). At this first, cognitive, stage it is good for the coach to give feedback (not too much though) about the outcome of successful practice. For instance, if the child plays a good backhand shot, ask them what the position of the grip was so they can make the connection.

The second, or associative, stage of learning is when children start to think less and less about the skill as some parts of the movement are memorised. The coach can tell when this happens, as they become more consistent with the skill and can be introduced to it under different conditions such as increasing the pace of the 'feed' for the backhand shot.

The final, autonomous, stage is where there is little thought given to the skill, as it almost feels like a reaction or reflex and comes naturally. This is an important stage in learning skills as the performer can concentrate on other things while doing it. For instance, while playing a backhand shot the performer can be watching for the position of their opponent, ready for the next shot. It is really useful for the coach to know when a child has reached the autonomous stage of a skill. The coach can check this by introducing a new skill linked to the skill being taught. For instance, if the skill being taught was to keep the angle of the racquet the same for all backhand drives, ask the performer to concentrate on the position of the front foot during the drive. If the performance of the first skill (angle of racquet) is affected, it is assumed that the skill isn't at the third stage of learning, so the coach should concentrate on only the first skill again. If the first skill isn't affected, the coach can move on to a new skill and so on.

Developing the athlete

One of the main problems facing most coaches is how and when to progress the performance of the young athlete as opposed to the child who is generally participating just for fun. For this reason, many National Governing Bodies (NGBs) in the UK have adopted a long-term athlete development (LTAD) model introduced by Bayli, focusing on encouraging young people to participate in sport, which then gives them the opportunity to improve their skills. As the title 'long-term' suggests, Bayli's model is used over a period of many years and is broken down into several stages. Table 3.8 shows an adaptation of this model, which consists of five stages as opposed to four in Bayli's original one.

Table 3.8 A long-term athlete development model

Stage	Age	Emphasis
Fundamentals (multi-skills)	6–8 (girls) 6–9 (boys)	● Try a wide range of fun activities ● Focus on multi-skills rather than sports-specific skills ● De-emphasise competition ● Use fun games to develop fitness components
Learning to train	8–11 (girls) 9–12 (boys)	● Focus on preferred activities ● Start to introduce competition ● Show how to train for the activity
Training to train	11–14 (girls) 12–15 (boys)	● Train in groups according to maturation ● Girls train separately from boys ● Avoid excessive high-impact ● Account for growth spurts
Training to compete	14–17 (girls) 15–18 (boys)	● Start to develop sports-specific skills and work on tactics ● Use specific fitness programmes to help achieve goals ● Be aware of overtraining and too many competitions at this stage
Training to win	17+ (girls) 18+ (boys)	● Training should now be programmed with respect to competition

The model in table 3.8 has been adapted to show five stages to be consistent with the Sports Coach UK model, which also uses five stages. It shows that, in the early years, children should be introduced to as many activities as possible that have a range of multi-skills and an emphasis on fun and play. Leading up to puberty and the start of growth spurts, a more specific emphasis should be put on the preferred activities of the child; competition should also be introduced. It should be noted here that the ages in the model are just a guide and coaches should be using the maturation age and not the chronological age. Once into the 'growth spurt' age range, the coach should be aware that performance of skills may decline as children struggle to cope with the rapidly increasing length of their limbs. This is also a particularly important time at which to limit excessive high-intensity impact training and to seek further advice for those children who are suffering from growing pains.

CHAPTER FOUR
Components of fitness

Objectives

After completing this chapter the reader should be able to:

- Define the term 'energy system' and discuss the systems available in the body in relation to exercise.
- Explain the impact on the energy systems during intermittent exercise.
- Identify components of fitness in relation to a variety of sports and activities.
- Discuss the benefits of training and guidelines in relation to cardiovascular endurance.
- Identify methods of measuring cardiovascular intensity levels.
- Discuss the benefits of training and guidelines in relation to muscular strength and endurance.
- Identify methods of measuring resistance intensity levels.
- Define the terms 'flexibility' and 'stability' and how they interact.
- List and describe different methods of stretching.
- Identify and describe the components of motor skills.
- List and briefly describe the factors that can affect components of fitness.
- Define the term 'overtraining' and describe ways in which to measure it.

Introduction

Before we look at the components of fitness, it would make sense to understand a little about the topic of energy systems – systems in the body that supply the energy needed for doing sport or activities, which we will call work. The description of energy systems in this chapter will be brief, as even an overview of this particular topic can be extremely huge and complicated, and therefore beyond the scope and purpose of this book. Should coaches wish to read more in-depth information relating to energy systems, they are referred to *The Advanced Fitness Instructor's Handbook* (Coulson and Archer, 2008).

Energy systems

Regardless of whether the body is at rest or moving during some kind of exercise, energy must always be supplied for chemical reactions to take place and to the muscles for movement to occur. The energy that is used in the body for muscles to contract is called 'adenosine triphosphate' (ATP) and is sometimes known as the 'energy currency' in the body. An ATP molecule is made up of the adenosine part with three ('tri' meaning three) phosphate groups bonded (this just means attached) to each other as in figure 4.1.

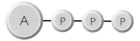

Fig. 4.1 A molecule of ATP

ATP is an amazing molecule as it can provide energy whenever one of the phosphates is broken off. In simple terms, the body can release enzymes to break off the phosphates from the store of ATP in the body, which in turn release an amount of energy, as can be seen in figure 4.2. This means, therefore, that the more ATP there is, the more phosphates can be broken off and the more energy can be released.

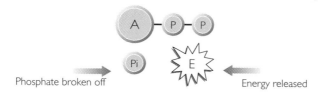

Phosphate broken off   Energy released

Fig. 4.2 A phosphate (Pi) broken off to release energy

Sources of ATP

The main problem with the store of ATP in the body being used for exercise is that there is only enough ATP in the body to last for about four seconds. For this reason, ATP has to be remade or provided in some way by other sources. Carbohydrates (pasta, rice, bread etc.), fats (butter, oils and in meat) and protein (mainly in meat) are all sources of food that can be digested to provide a large source of ATP.

Did you know
If we ran out of ATP in the body we would actually die.

In simple terms, foods release ATP once they have gone through the process of digestion. This process of food being used to provide ATP energy is occurring on a continuous basis in the body, but that depends on how much ATP is needed, which in turn depends on the amount of muscle contraction we do (in the form of the exercise carried out). Obviously when exercising at a higher intensity level, more ATP is needed to supply the energy demand. As a very general guide, carbohydrates are used mainly to supply ATP in the short term and fats are used mainly in the long term. Protein can be used but is usually only a standby source of ATP energy.

You may be familiar with the terms 'aerobic' and 'anaerobic' being applied to the exercise or activity that is being done. These terms, however, are related to the energy system that provides the ATP during the exercise. If the system used to provide ATP uses oxygen in the process, the exercise is known as 'aerobic'. If it does not use oxygen, the exercise is known as 'anaerobic'. It is commonly agreed that there are three systems within the body that are used to supply ATP: the ATP-PC system, the aerobic system and the anaerobic system.

- ATP-PC system: This system uses stores of a chemical called 'phospho-creatine' in the body to provide ATP. We will not be dealing with this system in detail, as it affects only the first few seconds of exercise before the other systems start to contribute.
- Aerobic system: In this system both carbohydrate and fat can be used as long as oxygen is available in the breakdown process. Lots more energy can be produced if fat is the main source providing the ATP.
- Anaerobic system: This system uses carbohydrate as the main food to produce ATP. One of the problems with doing this is that high levels of a chemical called 'lactic acid' can be produced, which eventually becomes uncomfortable (you may know this as the 'burn') and the exercise has to be reduced or stopped.

Did you know

During a 60-metre sprint an athlete will run almost the entire race using mainly the ATP-PC system.

Interaction of energy systems

It may seem strange, but our body uses all three of the energy systems at the same time – just in different amounts depending on what we are doing. For example, when we exercise, the intensity and duration of the exercise we are doing dictates which energy system will be used to supply the majority of the energy. This can be seen in figure 4.3, which shows how the aerobic and anaerobic systems interact during a bout of exercise.

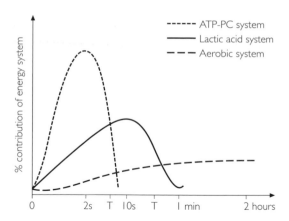

Fig. 4.3 Percentage contribution of energy systems over a short-term period

If we take the example of a session of low-intensity and long-duration exercise, we can see in figure 4.3 that, at the start of the exercise period (usually when we do a warm-up), the anaerobic system contributes more to energy production than does the aerobic system. As the exercise session continues beyond the duration of a few minutes, the contribution from the aerobic system increases to a point where, after several minutes (and at low to medium intensity), most of the energy is coming from the aerobic system and the contribution from the anaerobic system becomes much less as a result. However, it should also be noted that, towards the start of the exercise session, most of the ATP that is produced by the aerobic system comes from a source of carbohydrates, whereas once the exercise has been going for a reasonable amount of time (this depends on the fitness level of the individual and other things), most of the ATP then comes from various sources of fat stored in the body.

Did you know
A fitter person takes less time to get to the 'fat burning' stage than an unfit person!

Intermittent exercise

This particular situation is all fine and well if the exercise that is done stays at a low intensity; however, this is not usually the case with children, as they often have sudden bursts of high intensity (anaerobic) in most activities that they do. This type of exercise is known as 'intermittent'. If children do take part in intermittent activities, there is a sudden requirement for extra energy in order to cope with the high-intensity bursts. The extra energy in this case usually comes from the carbohydrate stores in the body. The problem with this is that if the burst of anaerobic exercise is high enough, large amounts of carbohydrate will be needed to provide the greater levels of energy required to sustain the high-intensity exercise. Recall from earlier in this chapter that lactic acid is produced during anaerobic exercise, so the bursts of high-intensity exercise cannot be sustained for very long or at too high an intensity level. It is generally found that high-intensity exercise producing large amounts of lactic acid can normally only be sustained for about two minutes (but much less in unfit people). Try doing the task in table 4.1, which shows the main energy systems used for typical sporting activities. Part of it has been already filled in – you just need to complete the rest.

Table 4.1 Main energy systems and various activities

TRY THIS

For each event or sport below, place a tick in the box corresponding to what you think is the main energy system used.

	ATP-PC	Aerobic (carbs)	Aerobic (fat)	Anaerobic
Triceps				
Marathon run				
60m sprint	✓			
400m sprint				✓
1500m run		✓		
Football match				
Tennis match				
50m swim				
1500m swim				
Tour de France cycle			✓	

Sometimes it is difficult to work out which is the main energy system being used during a particular event or activity. In this case the coach should not concern themselves too much about the particular energy systems but just try to replicate the demands of the event as closely as possible in training (*see* chapter 7).

Did you know
Plants also use ATP as a form of energy!

Components for sports and events
Most coaches associate training with the purpose of getting fitter; however, if you were to ask a number of coaches (or players for that matter) what being fit meant, you would probably get quite a lot of different answers. The problem with this is that, even if there was a common definition of 'fitness', not all coaches would agree with it. The term 'fitness', or to be more precise 'physical fitness', can be divided into several discrete areas, or 'components of fitness' as they are better known (*see* fig. 4.4).

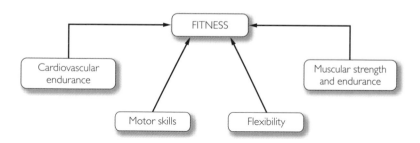

Fig. 4.4 Components of fitness

Each of these components can be trained for and be adapted individually without any of the others necessarily improving. Therefore, depending on the type of training carried out and the particular needs of the sport or event, an individual can be classed as 'fit' in one or more of the fitness components but not necessarily in them all. The components of physical fitness that we will cover in this book are cardiovascular endurance, muscular strength and endurance, flexibility and motor skills (of which there are several sub-components). Try completing the task in table 4.2 to identify which components of fitness you think are required for different sports.

Table 4.2 Components of fitness for sports and events

TRY THIS

For each sport or event below place a tick in the box or boxes corresponding to what you think are required components of fitness.

	Cardiovascular endurance	Muscular strength	Muscular endurance	Flexibility	Balance	Speed	Agility	Power
Snooker				✓	✓			
Rugby								
Sprinting								
Sprint cycle								
Darts								
Football			✓					
Tennis					✓		✓	
High jump								✓
800m swim								

Cardiovascular endurance

Quite often you will hear the term 'endurance training' as opposed to the term 'cardio-vascular endurance training' even though really they just mean the same thing (or they should do!). Cardiovascular endurance refers to the ability of the heart and lungs to deliver oxygen to the working muscles of the body (work aerobically) and for those muscles to use this oxygen in order to do work (exercise, sport, events, activities etc.). It is obvious, therefore, that oxygen is very important in the process of providing the body with energy. Cardiovascular endurance is something that is measured very often using various types of fitness test, such as the multi-stage fitness test, which all measure the amount of oxygen the body is able to deliver. Regardless of the test of cardiovas-cular endurance being done, any one of them can result in a measurement called 'volume of oxygen' (VO_2), with VO_2max being the maximum amount of oxygen that can be delivered to the working muscles. It makes sense therefore that the more oxygen a person can get to their muscles the more exercise they will be able to do.

Did you know

The units used to measure VO_2 are millilitres of oxygen per kilo-gram of bodyweight per minute. This is written as – $mlO_2.kg^{-1}min^{-1}$.

Benefits of training

Associated with undertaking regular sessions of cardiovascular training are many published benefits, which include both physiological and psychological areas. Figure 4.5 shows just some of the many benefits.

When trying to prescribe cardiovascular training, however, the volume, intensity and

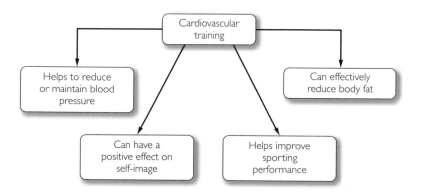

Fig. 4.5 Benefits of cardiovascular training

frequency of the activities has to be taken into consideration as they play an important role with respect to improvement, overtraining and prevention of injury.

VOLUME

'Cardiovascular training volume' is just another term for the amount of cardiovascular exercise or activity done and is normally measured by mileage or time. Sometimes the coach might not know the distance being covered, so they might prefer to prescribe the training by using duration. For instance, the coach might set a training programme that has three 5-kilometre runs each week or he might set three 30-minute runs each week. Be aware, though, that team game players will be covering up to several kilometres each during the course of a match.

Did you know

Premiership football players can cover more than 15 kilometres in a game!

INTENSITY

The term 'intensity' simply refers to 'how hard' the exercise or activity is: in other words, in the case of cardiovascular endurance, how hard it would be to cycle or run at a particular pace. As the intensity of the exercise increases (this can be running faster, cycling uphill etc.), the amount of oxygen required to cope with the demand of the exercise also increases, and therefore, to get more oxygen around the body, the heart rate increases in proportion. This increase in heart rate due to an increase in exercise intensity is known as a 'linear relationship'. In other words, if intensity was steadily increased

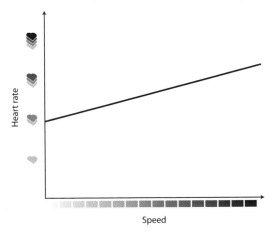

Fig. 4.6 Relationship between heart rate and speed

and heart rate measured after each increase, the points on the graph would fall close to a straight line as can be seen in figure 4.6.

This linear relationship between heart rate and intensity is really useful for tracking fitness levels. For instance, if a test is set up to measure the heart rate of a performer after increasing the speed during a run, this is known as taking a 'baseline' (pre-training) measurement. If the same test is done several weeks later and the measurement line is lower (as seen in fig. 4.7), this indicates that the performer is fitter as they are able to maintain the same speed at a lower heart rate.

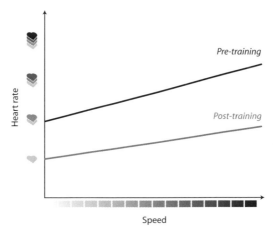

Fig. 4.7 Relationship between heart rate and speed for pre- and post-training

One of the problems associated with children doing aerobic sessions with short bursts of higher intensity exercise is that it is difficult for the coach to monitor all the children in the session in order to judge how hard they are working. There are many different ways in which to monitor the work rate or intensity, such as by the performers wearing monitors that track their heart rates, but in a group situation the RPE scale is probably the most useful tool. RPE stands for 'rate of perceived exertion', which simply means how hard you think you are working. The original RPE scale was developed by Dr. Gunnar Borg for adults but has since been adapted and modified for children as shown in figure 4.8.

Intensity	Explanation
0-rest	How you feel when sitting or resting
1-easy	Light walking; no sweating
2-pretty hard	Playing and just starting to sweat
3-harder	Playing hard and sweating
4-hard	Running hard; sweating a lot
5-maximal	Hardest you have ever worked; ready to collapse

Fig. 4.8 Typical 5-point RPE scale adapted for children

The RPE scale is designed to be as user-friendly as possible. It can be used by showing the scale to the children who are participating in the activity session and then asking them what intensity number they think they are at on the scale. The scale itself is not always a useful one for younger children as they have difficulty visualising what the words mean. A more visual, cartoon-like scale could always be designed relevant to the age of the children you are coaching. Figure 4.9 gives a typical example of a scale used with younger children. Depending on the response, the coach can adapt the session to keep the participants

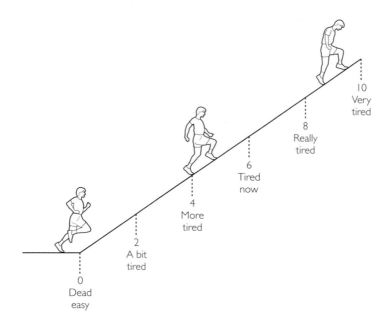

Fig. 4.9 Typical 10-point visual RPE scale for younger children

at the level that has been planned. For instance, a coach might want to do a warm-up where the level goes up to 1 or 2, but then increase the intensity to 3 for the main session interspersed with 4 for brief periods of time, and back down to 1 for the cool-down. Constant checking of where the participants feel they are at is required, which means that sessions should be flexible. The coach might find this system difficult to use at first but it soon becomes easier with practice.

FREQUENCY

'Frequency' is a term that simply means 'how often' the exercise or activity takes place. For example, a coach might have three training sessions per week but only do cardiovascular training in two of them; therefore, the frequency of training is three times per week but the frequency of cardiovascular training is twice per week. The coach must be aware that most of the published guidelines about exercise or activity relate to the frequency of the specific component of fitness and not generally to the number of activity or exercise sessions.

Muscular strength and endurance

The terms 'muscular strength' and 'muscular endurance' both relate to components of fitness that can be trained independently. For example, a person can have good muscular strength but poor muscular endurance, or vice versa. The difference between muscular strength and muscular endurance is not always easy to describe or explain in terms of resistance training.

The particular definitions suggest that muscular strength relates to training with heavy weights and doing few repetitions, whereas muscular endurance is related to training with lighter weights but doing a higher number of repetitions.

Benefits of training

Like all other components of fitness, resistance training has many benefits, such as those outlined in figure 4.10. Research shows that strain, as a result of resistance

> **Definition**
> ● 'Muscular strength' can be described as the maximum amount of force a muscle or muscle group can generate.
> ● 'Muscular endurance' can be described as the ability of a muscle or muscle group to perform repeated contractions against a resistance over a period of time.

training, can help stimulate bone growth, which would obviously help to protect against breaks. It has also shown that muscular strength can help to prevent muscle strains. Particular sports or events would also benefit from an increase in muscular strength and endurance as these are important components of fitness in almost all activities. As for cardiovascular training, the volume, intensity and frequency of exercise also have to be taken into consideration when prescribing resistance training, since they can also play an important role with respect to performance improvement, overtraining and injury prevention.

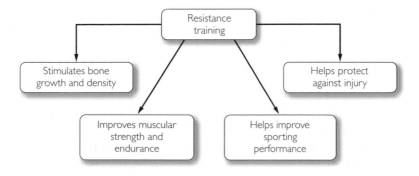

Fig. 4.10 Benefits of resistance training

VOLUME

The volume in relation to resistance training can be measured in two ways:

1. Sets × Repetitions
2. Sets × Repetitions × Load

The 'load' is just the amount of weight lifted, the 'repetitions' is the number of times the weight is lifted and 'sets' just refers to how many times this is repeated. For example, for an individual who performs 3 sets of 10 repetitions with 80kg, the volume can be calculated either as 30 repetitions (at 80kg) or as 2400kg.

INTENSITY

Training intensity (otherwise known as the 'load') is just the amount of weight to be lifted. Published guidelines often refer to what is known as 'repetition maximum' (RM), which simply means the maximum weight that can be lifted for a specific number of repetitions. For example, if a guideline states that the performer should train with 10RM loads, then this is the maximum weight that can be lifted by the performer for 10 repetitions. Intensity can also be expressed as a percentage of the maximum weight that an individual can lift (1RM). For example, you will often see a statement such as 'train with loads of 80% of 1RM'. This just means 80% of the maximum that a performer can lift. The problem with this method is that it means individuals need to find out their maximum capability, which is not recommended for children.

FREQUENCY

This is exactly the same as for cardiovascular endurance but relates to how many times a week you train with weights instead. Be aware, though, that this also refers to muscles being trained and not just to the training sessions. For example, an individual might do three training sessions a week but only train a particular muscle (chest for instance) once: the training frequency for the chest is therefore once per week.

Resistance training is sometimes associated with an increase in muscle size (cross-sectional area), which is called 'hypertrophy', although this is not as easy to achieve as some people might think. In order to gain considerable muscle size, there are many factors that must be considered. Some of these factors for an individual include their genetics needing to be right (a good proportion of fast-twitch fibres in the muscles); the need to train hard using weights that are appropriate; and their nutrition having to be good enough to support the training and to help protein re-synthesis.

Definition

'Re-synthesis' is a term that is used to describe what happens when protein breaks down then rebuilds again.

With resistance training, it is also common for individuals to experience, in the days following a training session, a sensation of pain or stiffness in the muscles that have been trained. This sensation of pain or stiffness is called 'delayed onset of muscle soreness' (DOMS). Coaches, therefore, should advise participants to do some light aerobic exercise, such as brisk walking or cycling, following resistance training as it is thought to reduce DOMS.

Flexibility

It is common for the terms flexibility and stretching to be used interchangeably, but they shouldn't as they are very different in description. 'Flexibility' is often defined as 'the ability to move a joint through its complete range of motion'. It can be seen from the definition that flexibility is an ability that someone has, whereas 'stretching' is a term that relates to training, as described in the definition 'an exercise done to either maintain or improve flexibility'. Flexibility is known as 'joint-specific' in that an individual may be flexible in one joint and not necessarily in another. Although over-flexibility is related to the possibility of joint instability and injury, one of the main benefits of maintaining a reasonable range of motion of the joints is to allow individuals to carry out daily activities as long as possible throughout their lives. As some sports require a greater than normal amount of flexibility, those athletes are usually willing to accept the greater risk of joint injury in later life.

Did you know

Many Japanese desk workers stand up every hour to stretch. This can improve the flexibility of the hip-flexor muscles, which if left in a shortened seated position all day can contribute to back pain.

Stability

For reasons of risk of joint injury, it is difficult to talk about flexibility without having some understanding of stability. The term 'stability' is really the opposite of flexibility in that it refers to how joints can be kept in position to do the job they were designed to do. For instance, the shoulder joint is much more flexible than the hip joint because, even though they are both 'ball and socket' joints, the hip joint is much deeper than the shoulder joint. This is because the hip joint requires a great deal more stability than the shoulder joint for everyday use, and also requires a greater range of motion and flexibility to move.

Flexibility beyond a 'normal' range of motion may be useful or necessary for certain sports but, for the purpose of joint stability, it should be remembered that the muscular system is considered to be one of the three main systems that contribute to joint stability, as can be seen in figure 4.11. All three systems are widely accepted to be of major importance in the prevention of injury mainly as a result of joint instability. As ligament tissue is prone to tearing, the muscular system is often required to provide a greater amount of stability for joints, especially during dynamic movements. In many cases where the flexibility of an individual is considered to be beyond the normal range of motion (often referred to as 'hyperflexibility'), joint stability is often lacking or reduced, which can result in a variety of conditions of joint injury. In cases where the range of

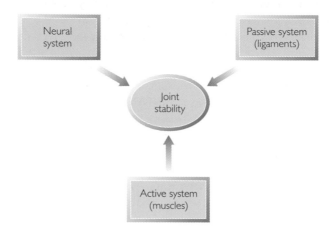

Fig. 4.11 Systems contributing to overall joint stability

flexibility of an individual is considered to be less than normal, injury such as muscle strain can occur.

Types of stretch

Although it is often stated that stretching can help prevent injury, there is little evidence to support this. It has been shown that both a high degree of flexibility and a low degree of flexibility can increase injury risk. It is recommended that people with tight muscles would probably benefit most from stretching, whereas people who are natur-ally supple should not engage in more than light stretching. The most effective stretching occurs when the muscles are warm and there are many types that can be used, including static, dynamic, ballistic and PNF.

- Static: This is when a stretch is performed and held for a period of time at a point of mild tension (not pain). The point of tension is a subjective perception (what the person feels) and is thought to reduce as the person gets used to stretching. If a static stretch is held long enough, this tension usually subsides and the stretch can be taken further if required. If a partner or another group of muscles assists in the stretching process, it is called an 'active' stretch. If there is no assistance in the stretch it is called a 'passive' stretch.

- Dynamic: This relates to stretching in motion where an agonist muscle is contracted to stretch an antagonist muscle (the muscle doing the work contracts to stretch the opposite muscle). This type of stretching is usually carried out in a slow and controlled manner in order to minimise the risk of injury and to mimic the types of movement that may be used in the exercises to follow.
- Ballistic: This is where bouncing movements are caused by momentum or gravity. This type of stretching is usually carried out by athletes who are familiar with it. As there is little control of the movement through muscular contraction, there is a greater risk of injury.
- PNF: Proprioceptive neuromuscular facilitation, commonly known as 'PNF' (you can see why it is shortened to PNF!), is a type of partner-assisted stretching, usually carried out on tight or injured muscles. There is usually a degree of training associated with this type of stretching and so it should only be performed by those who are qualified. Contract-relax-antagonist-contract (CRAC) is one form of PNF.

It is impossible for any individual to have what can be considered to be optimum flexibility in all joints, as the demands of sports are so different. It is the job of the coach, therefore, to identify how much and in what specific joints flexibility is required for the particular sport or event and then to plan a programme of stretching exercises to suit. The task in table 4.3 should help the coach to think about the process of understanding the demands of various sports or events in relation to the flexibility required for them. Coaches will, however, need to assess the level of flexibility with their players. As this is beyond the scope of this book, coaches are recommended to refer to *Practical Fitness Testing* (Coulson and Archer, 2009) for a comprehensive guide to testing components of fitness.

If the coach feels that a child is particularly inflexible and that they are not becoming more flexible with their normal stretching exercises, they should always refer this case to an appropriate specialist, rather than just leave the child to cope with the demands of the sport or event in which they are participating.

Motor skills

The term 'motor skills' is dealt with in more detail in other chapters; however, for the purpose of this chapter we will deal with motor skills as though it was not a single component. There are many sub-components, such as balance, speed, agility and power, associated with motor skills and these will be different depending on the source of information. All the sub-component areas can be improved with training. Table 4.4 gives a brief definition of each sub-component.

Table 4.3 Flexibility requirements for various sports and events

TRY THIS!
Place a tick in the box that is relevant to each sport in terms of the importance of flexibility.

	Low	Medium	High
Football		✓	
Rugby			
Netball			
Basketball			
Darts			
Snooker			
Cycling			
Badminton			
Tennis			
Archery	✓		
Karate			✓
Judo			
Showjumping			

Balance

Generally speaking there are two types or categories relating to balance, both of which can be developed with the correct type of training, especially in young children. The categories are known as 'static' and 'dynamic' balance and, as the names imply, they are reasonably straightforward to describe.

Table 4.4 Sub-components of motor skills

Sub-component	Description
Balance	This is the ability to maintain equilibrium at all times. Proprioceptors (sensors) in the body, as well as the inner ear (vestibular) and the eyes, give information to the brain on the position of all limbs.
Speed	This can be improved through muscle coordination, efficient body movement, core strength and flexibility.
Agility	This is the ability to change direction at speed.
Power	This combines strength and speed and can be developed through plyometric (stretch-rebound) and resistance training.

- 'Static' balance is simply maintaining equilibrium (balance) in a stationary position.
- 'Dynamic' balance is maintaining equilibrium while in motion.

The ability of an individual to be able to balance is absolutely fundamental to any effective movement, not just in a sporting context but also in everyday life. For example, when walking, jogging or running in a straight line, balance is absolutely crucial for effective foot placement, body control and reduction of 'core' movement. For this reason, balance is also often described as 'control of the centre of mass' because if we are in control of our centre of mass, we are in a balanced and stable position. Although a complex area, there are systems in the body that contribute to balance: the proprioceptive, visual and vestibular systems are considered to be the main ones.

Definition
'Proprioceptors' are tiny sensors in the body that detect tension in tendons. This information is relayed to the brain and can be used to work out the position of joints.

PROPRIOCEPTIVE SYSTEM
Throughout the joints of the body there are tiny sensors known as 'proprioceptors'. These sensors are able to send information to the brain regarding the exact position

of the joints on an ongoing basis so that the position of all the limbs is regularly updated for balance purposes. For instance, if you were going over on your ankle, the proprioceptors would send information to the brain to say the ankle joint was not in a good position: in response, the brain would stimulate the necessary leg muscles to regain balance.

VISUAL SYSTEM

Most of our balance information comes from what we see – in other words from our visual referencing system. Our eyes use the objects around us to determine our balance; the following example can illustrate how much we rely on this. Have you ever been running on a treadmill, then when it stops you feel like you are still moving? This is because when you walk or run normally, the image on the retina from objects around you changes size as you get nearer or further away. When you are on a treadmill, the objects around you don't change size and this causes confusion in the brain!

VESTIBULAR SYSTEM

Within the inner ear there are a series of canals filled with fluid. The canals are lined with tiny hairs and if we move in any direction, the fluid flows over the tiny hairs, which provide information to the brain that we are moving (in a particular direction). This is why your balance can be affected if you ever get an ear infection: vertigo is caused by an ear infection that can lead to loss of balance.

The brain relies upon information from the eyes, ears and proprioceptors for balance purposes. Through training of these systems, the ability to perform balance skills usually becomes more effective. In addition, it is thought that the brain becomes more able to interpret the balance information from the various systems so that it can make the appropriate movement response. The communication system within the body (made up of nerves) is developed during movement skills training. The 'neural networks' within the brain and nervous system become more extensive as more and more neural links are created through repetition of movement skills. When complex movements are introduced, the requirements of balance are increased. The need to land, accelerate, change direction or decelerate requires advanced balance skills. A training programme, therefore, should follow a logical progression, in relation to the complexity of skills to be performed, that will allow the development of balance skills.

Speed

The term 'speed' can mean different things to different people depending on the context in which it is being used. For instance, in sprinting (or any sport in which there is sprinting involved), speed could be described as 'the time taken to go between two points'. In sports such as boxing or martial arts, however, speed can refer to how fast a punch or a kick can be thrown (or how fast a punch or kick can be avoided). In whatever context though, there is normally a reaction to something (known as a 'stimulus') before a movement at speed occurs. If we take the case of sprinting, it is not as simple as we might first think, as it can contain several phases depending on the distance of the sprint.

As can be seen in figure 4.12, it is normal for most athletic sprint distances to contain a reaction (to a stimulus) phase, acceleration phase, maximal speed phase and speed maintenance/deceleration phase. However, in most team sports such as soccer, rugby, basketball, netball and hockey, the typical sprint distances covered during a game are generally only between 10 and 20 metres, which means that maximal speed is not really achieved, as players can take about 30 metres to reach it. In team sports, therefore, reacting quickly and accelerating into position rapidly is often more important than achieving maximal speed.

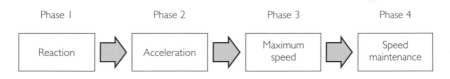

Fig. 4.12 Phases of a sprint

REACTION PHASE

As mentioned previously, before any movement can take place, a player must be able to identify and react to a particular stimulus. This is known as 'reaction time'. Depending on the sport or event, the stimulus could take many forms such as the movement of a ball, the reaction to an opponent or opportunity in a game situation, or simply the gun going off at the start of a track race. It is thought (and has often been demonstrated) that reaction times can be improved as a result of regular training. Reaction times in general sporting situations are typically measured to be in the region of 100–200 milliseconds (0.1–0.2s).

ACCELERATION PHASE

In this phase, the term 'acceleration' is simply used to describe an increase or a change in the speed of a player. In this phase of sprinting there tends to be a rapid increase in the number of steps taken in a given time period (this is known as the 'stride frequency') and a steadier increase in the length of the stride that is taken. Stride length and stride frequency are terms that are often used (and elements that are often trained) by sprint coaches, and can be described and measured using the formulae:

$$\text{Stride length} = \frac{\text{Distance covered}}{\text{Number of strides}}$$

$$\text{Stride frequency} = \frac{\text{Number of strides}}{\text{Time taken}}$$

MAXIMAL SPEED PHASE (30–80M)

Highly trained or elite-level sprinters usually reach their individual maximal speed at distances of approximately 50-60 metres, whereas in less trained individuals, maximal speed is normally reached after approximately 30 metres. For this reason, the maximal speed phase of sprinting plays only a minor role in many team sports. This is because it is rare that a player is allowed to run for more than 20-30 metres during a game situation.

In this phase a player would have a more upright running position, as opposed to leaning forwards in the acceleration phase. The hamstrings (muscles at the back of the thigh) are considered to be a more important muscle group during the maximal speed phase, due to the cycle-like motion in which they play a major role. This means, therefore, that hamstring strength and flexibility are important for sprinting.

SPEED MAINTENANCE/DECELERATION PHASE

Trying to maintain maximal speed beyond 80 metres is really difficult for most sprinters (unless you happen to be Usain Bolt). Once at maximal speed, a sprinter needs to be strong as fatigue and tiredness can cause the sprinter to slow down, which is known as 'deceleration'. It makes sense, therefore, that the more a person is sprint-trained the longer it will be before the deceleration phase begins.

Did you know?
Humans can reach speeds of up to 8km/hr in water, compared to fish, which can reach 108km/hr!

Depending on the sport, playing position or event and phase of the season, there may be a different requirement in terms of distances covered and typical recovery duration between sprints. Therefore, the coach must be able to identify and plan in areas such as distance, intensity, recovery and volume.

DISTANCE

The design of a training programme for speed depends mainly on the training goal such as improving acceleration, maximal speed or conditioning. For acceleration (most relevant for team sports as mentioned earlier), the training distances should be relatively short (in the region of 10–30 metres). When training for maximal speed, as in sprinting or sports such as rugby or Gaelic football, the distances should be from 40 to 80 metres since maximum speed is in most cases only reached between 30 and 60 metres. For conditioning training, depending on the individual, longer sprints of from 80 to 400 metres may be required.

INTENSITY
The intensity of a training session can be set in many ways, for instance by using a percentage of the player's current personal best (PB) over the required distance (e.g. 90% of their 60-metre PB). The intensity can also be set by using self-perception, for example an 80% maximal effort. With regular practice, players should become more accurate in estimating their effort – an RPE scale could be used for this. In order to run faster, individuals must train fast and much of the training must be at maximal speed. Therefore, coaches often vary the pace of the training sprints, alternating between full-effort and speed-maintenance phases (e.g. first 40 metres all-out, next 20 metres maintain speed, then 20 metres all-out). This type of training is known as 'ins and outs'.

RECOVERY
There are many things that can affect how much recovery is needed between training sessions and this makes it difficult for the coach to deal with it. Also, the duration of the recovery allowed between sprint repetitions within a training session is vital as it can affect the intensity of the next sprint in that session. For example, 100-metre sprinters may take from five to ten minutes to recover between sprints. In most sports, however, the recovery duration is not fixed and the individual must perform a repeated sprint when required. In professional soccer, for example, typical recovery durations are one minute on average and in rugby they range from two to four minutes for certain playing positions.

VOLUME
As with all training, care must be taken that the volume of training for children is not excessive as it may result not only in negative effects on performance but also in injury. The number of speed sessions per week often depends on the nature of the sport or event being trained for. For instance, individuals who participate in team sports will usually benefit most from two to three sprint training sessions per week, whereas a specialist sprinter often performs up to six sprint training sessions per week. In order to avoid over-training, coaches often stipulate that different aspects of sprint training must be done within a certain training period. For example, an acceleration training session can be undertaken on a particular day, followed by a maximal speed session the next day.

Agility
It is difficult to find a precise definition of agility (often interchanged with the word 'quickness') as the definition varies depending on the source. 'Agility' is commonly

defined as 'a rapid whole-body movement with change of velocity or direction in response to a stimulus'. This definition implies that a person needs physical qualities such as strength and power to be able to move rapidly and also have the ability to anticipate. If we take the example of a sporting activity, agility can refer to a player being able to stop, start and change direction as quickly as possible. For this reason, it is thought that agility is made up of several fitness components such as balance, coordination, strength and power. Agility can also be thought of in two ways: as programmed and random (depending on the situation and the sport).

- 'Programmed agility' refers to a movement that is agile but does not involve the reaction to a stimulus. Take the example of a high-jumper who needs to be agile enough to take off at a different angle to the approach run. The athlete has calculated the direction of the movement and has not needed to change this in response to any external stimulus.
- 'Random agility' refers to a movement that is agile and does involve the reaction to a stimulus. Take the example of the goalkeeper who reacts to a well-struck volley that is heading for the far corner but then takes a deflection. After starting to move in one direction the goalkeeper is agile enough to change body position quickly in order to make the save.

For the task in table 4.5, note how important you think the agility requirements are for different sports.

Power

When we talk about the power of a player, we are usually referring to some sort of strength capability. This makes sense because a simple description of power could be 'strength at speed', although there are many more complex and scientific descriptions. Players in sports such as judo and rugby would often be referred to as powerful since they engage in physical contests in which, to be successful, they need a good strength base. In scientific terms, 'power' is usually measured in units of watts (W) and calculated using the formula:

$$\text{Power (W)} = \text{Force (kg.m.s}^{-2}) \times \text{Distance (m)} \div \text{Time (s)}$$

So in order to calculate the power that is created during a sport or event we need to know the force, the distance moved and the time taken. For instance, if we use the example of moving or lifting a weight, power is measured as the amount of weight that can be lifted or moved a certain distance in a certain amount of time. As you will have

Table 4.5 Agility requirements for various sports and events

	Low	Medium	High
Football			✓
100m sprint			
Netball			
Hammer throw			
Darts			
Snooker			
Cycling			
Badminton			
Tennis			
Archery	✓		
Karate			✓
Judo			

noticed in the formula for power, however, we need force and not weight. To convert the weight to force we simply multiply the weight by the value $9.81 m.s^{-2}$, which then gives us the force.

Once we have calculated the force, we just need to measure the distance travelled in metres and time how long the movement took. The first example illustrates this:

Example 1: Calculating the power of an athlete during a movement

Imagine a sumo wrestling contest in which one of the players pushes the other one backwards. If the player being pushed backwards weighs 140kg, the distance moved is 2m and the push took 0.5s, the power can be calculated as follows:

Power = Force × Distance ÷ Time
     = (Weight × 9.81) × Distance ÷ Time

Putting the values in we get:

Power = (140 × 9.81) × 2 ÷ 0.5 = 5493.6W

However, we can see in the formula that the faster the lift or movement of the weight, the greater the power that will be generated (assuming the weight and distance stay the same). This can be seen in the next example, in which the sumo wrestler decides to push harder and takes only 0.25 seconds as opposed to 0.5 seconds. The power generated as a result has almost doubled.

Example 2: Calculating the power with a harder push

In the same sumo wrestling contest but the push now taking 0.25s, the power can be calculated as follows:

Power = (Weight × 9.81) × Distance ÷ Time

Putting the values in we get:

Power = (140 × 9.81) × 2 ÷ 0.25 = 10,987.2W

You will often find that power is written as 'power output' as it usually refers to a specific period of time or to a specific skill performed. For the second example, therefore, we could say that the sumo wrestler has a power output of 10,987.2 watts when pushing his opponent backwards. When using different loads or weights, the power output that is developed will also change as a result. The third example of the sumo wrestler shows the calculation of the power output, but this time with an opponent weighing only 120 kilograms.

It makes sense that the speed of movement would probably be faster (in the example,

Example 3: Calculating the power with a different load

If the player being pushed back now weighs 120kg, the distance moved is 2m and the push took 0.2s the power can be calculated as follows:

Power = (Weight × 9.81) × Distance ÷ Time

Putting the values in we get:

Power = (120 × 9.81) × 2 ÷ 0.2 = 11,772W

0.2s as opposed to 0.25s) if the load being moved was lighter. The example shows that the lighter the load the more the power output could be (generally speaking), due to the length of time required to move the load through the full movement being shorter. So in simple terms, power depends on the strength of the athlete, the load and the speed at which the load is moved over a certain distance.

Factors that affect components of fitness

There are many factors that can affect the fitness (components of fitness to be precise) of children. Some of these factors can have an immediate effect and others will have more of a long-term effect. We have no control over some of them, such as body type, gender and age, whereas other factors, such as fitness level, lifestyle and environment, we can have some control over.

Body type

As mentioned previously in chapter 2, the distribution of different types of fibre within muscles is determined at birth and can only be affected slightly with training. Therefore, the old saying 'we are what we are born with' is essentially true. A person born with a higher percentage distribution of fast-twitch fibres will obviously be more predisposed to strength-type events, whereas a person born with a high percentage of slow-twitch fibres will be predisposed to endurance-type events.

It is possible sometimes, judging by their body shape and size, to get an indication of the type of athlete someone could be. For instance, in relation to the overall shape of an individual there are three extreme classifications of body type that can be used: endo-morph, ectomorph and mesomorph. An 'endomorph' tends to excel at sports such as shot-put or discus, an 'ectomorph' tends to do well at endurance sports or events and a 'mesomorph' does well at sports such as rugby or boxing. It is common, however, for individuals to be more than one type and so a grading system for each classification can be used, but this is beyond the scope of this book. A description of the three clas-sifications of body type can be seen in table 4.6.

Table 4.6 Body type classifications

Endomorph	<ul><li>A pear-shaped body</li><li>A rounded head</li><li>Wide hips and shoulders</li><li>Wider front to back than side to side</li><li>A lot of fat on the body, upper arms and thighs</li></ul>
Ectomorph	<ul><li>A high forehead</li><li>Receding chin</li><li>Narrow shoulders and hips</li><li>A narrow chest and abdomen</li><li>Thin arms and legs</li><li>Little muscle and fat</li></ul>
Mesomorph	<ul><li>A wedge-shaped body</li><li>A cubical head</li><li>Wide broad shoulders</li><li>Muscled arms and legs</li><li>Narrow hips</li><li>Wider side to side than front to back</li></ul>

Gender

Even though the term 'gender' simply relates to being either a male or a female, it is becoming more common that female athletes are starting to show certain male characteristics (take the example of the embarrassing enquiry and aftermath of the 2009 World Athletic Championships with the South African women's 800-metre winner) that can make the task of identifying gender a very delicate one.

Did you know

In December 2006, 25-year-old Santhi Soundarajan from India was stripped of her silver medal for the 800-metre race in the Asian Games after failing a gender test.

Even though the subject is more complex than first imagined, it is well known that gender can have an important bearing on certain components of fitness. For example, cardiovascular potential (VO_2max as we know it) is typically about 15–30% lower in females than in males. Generally speaking, men are also capable of greater muscle hypertrophy. This is as a result of strength-training capabilities, as men tend to have a greater proportion of fast-twitch fibres and greater levels of hormones that affect growth. Also, as a general rule, women tend to be more flexible than men for childbirth purposes. Because of the differences in capabilities between men and women, there are very few sports or events where men compete against women.

Age

Another factor affecting fitness that we don't have control over is age. The process of ageing can have the effect of decreasing the level of the individual components of fitness; however, with children this doesn't really apply, as the components of fitness are developing throughout childhood and do not usually diminish until later in life. A common example of this is flexibility, which can be lost very quickly once a person reaches adulthood. This is not to say that we can't do anything about it, as there are many older individuals who retain flexibility by participating in exercises such as yoga and Pilates. Another effect of ageing is what we call 'osteoporosis', which is a weakening of the bones. Resistance training and generally keeping fit can help to reduce the risk of developing this condition.

Fitness level

One of the factors affecting the components of fitness that we can have any degree of control over is actual fitness level. Generally speaking, a less fit individual will initially make greater improvements in any of the components of fitness than a fitter person, as long as the training for that component of fitness is done correctly. This should be taken into account when setting goals and targets for individuals (*see* chapter 7).

Lifestyle

There are many aspects of lifestyle which we can control that can affect some of the components of fitness. One of the main areas related to lifestyle these days is psychological stress. Coaches shouldn't ever assume that children do not suffer from any effects of stress, as they commonly do so for various reasons. Stress is something that can have a detrimental effect on the way in which individuals can train and hence on the components of fitness.

Another area related to lifestyle that we can control is sleep. Many coaches underestimate the importance of sleep and how this can ultimately affect the child. There are many processes that occur during sleep, including the growth of bones and muscles as well as the repair of injuries. It is difficult as a coach to recognise the symptoms of lack of sleep because they range from irritability and sluggishness to hyperactivity. Coaches can only advise parents on children getting enough sleep but it is difficult to know how much sleep is actually needed. As a general guide, about 11 hours for younger children reducing to 9 hours for older children is often recommended. Remember, though, that too much sleep can also be a problem. See the top tips in table 4.7 for guidelines relating to children and sleep.

Table 4.7 Top tips for guidelines relating to children and sleep

1 Don't forget that it might take up to 30 minutes before children get to sleep so allow for this.

2 Try not to let children watch TV or play computer games before going to bed as this will make it more difficult to sleep.

3 Stick to a routine. Try to put children to bed at the same time each night.

4 Try not to let children eat at least two hours before going to bed if you can avoid it.

5 Children should avoid drinks containing caffeine before going to bed (chocolate, cocoa, coffee, tea, cola).

6 If children exercise during the day as often as possible, this should help them to sleep better.

Environment

One of the by-products of muscle contraction is heat: exercise or activity can warm the body. Children are not as efficient as adults at regulating body temperature so care must be taken in both cold and hot environments. Children tend to heat up very quickly in hot environments because their sweat glands produce much less sweat than adults, which means they don't cool down as quickly. This may be useful in a cooler environment but if they continue to heat up in a warm environment they can overheat, which is called 'hyperthermia' (taken from the Greek 'hyper' meaning 'more than', and 'therm' meaning 'heat'). This condition is serious and could lead to dehydration and heat exhaustion if not dealt with promptly. As this can happen quite frequently, and quickly in some cases, the coach must be aware of the signs of possible overheating and the precautions that can be put in place to minimise the risk (see table 4.8).

The effects of dehydration in children can be quite severe compared to adults as the more dehydrated the child becomes, the quicker they tend to heat up and overheat. It is extremely important, therefore, that children drink water at least every 10–15 minutes in warm environments (and also in cold environments) in order to prevent dehydration.

In cold environments children lose heat very quickly for many different reasons. Hypothermia (from the Greek 'hypo' meaning 'less than', and 'therm' meaning 'heat') is the term given to excessive loss of body temperature. Again, this is a serious condition that can lead to irregular heartbeats and even death, so correct clothing is absolutely vital in cold conditions.

Table 4.8 Signs of overheating and precautions

Overheating signs	Precautions
• Excessive sweating • Muscle cramps • Cold clammy skin • Loss of coordination • Dizziness and faintness • Very flushed skin • Nauseousness	• Always have water breaks before, during and after sessions • Use light coloured, gortex-type clothing • Use sunscreen • Limit duration of activities • Set up sessions in the shade if possible

Just as in the case of hyperthermia, the coach must be aware of the signs of possible overcooling and the precautions that can be put in place to minimise the risk (*see* table 4.9). Children react very quickly to environmental temperature so the coach must always be vigilant.

Table 4.9 Signs of overcooling and precautions

Overcooling signs	Precautions
• Excessive shivering • Very pale skin • Unable to talk clearly • Limited movements	• Always dress appropriately • Limit the duration of the session • Do a long warm-up • Keep all participants as active as possible • Drink water since dehydration can also occur

Overtraining

The term 'overtraining' is often used by coaches but is sometimes misunderstood. The term 'overreaching' may be used to mean the same thing but they are different terms. 'Overreaching' is thought to be excessive amounts of training that eventually leads to a condition of overtraining. Although difficult to describe, like many terms, 'overtraining' is understood as relating to physiological and/or psychological problems brought about by an excessive amount of training. Whether overtraining exists or not (this is a debate currently going on in science), it is an important area to be familiar with.

Problems with overtraining tend to be grouped into three areas: movement or co-ordination, physiological and psychological. Overtraining is not just a potential problem for athletes, as it can affect any child who participates in excessive amounts of activity. Many coaches find it difficult to deal with overtraining, as it is hard to diagnose. This is a valid point but there are potential signs that they could try to be aware of and look out for, some of which are described in table 4.10.

Many children suffer as a consequence of overtraining (and this can be for a variety of reasons). Sometimes the coach just does not recognise or is not aware of the symptoms as they appear, because they are too focused on the training or competitions. At other times, the coach might notice some of the symptoms starting to appear but is not convinced that they are due to overtraining. As soon as any overtraining symptoms are noticed, however, coaches should reduce the amount of training until the individual has recovered enough to recommence training. This is a difficult thing to do for many coaches, but with children it is especially important as it is always best to be cautious rather than run the risk of injury due to overtraining.

Table 4.10 Typical signs of overtraining

Problem area	Description
Movement or coordination	● More frequent (than usual) coordination problems ● Loses concentration more often than usual ● More difficulty trying to correct technique or skills
Physiological	● Decrease in cardio endurance ● Decrease in strength performance ● Decrease in speed performance
Psychological	● Sudden dislike for competition ● Suddenly starts using different tactics to normal ● Has a negative attitude and starts giving up easily ● Behaviour becomes difficult and sometimes obstructive ● Becomes anxious and depressed ● Appears to lack any sort of motivation ● Starts becoming introvert

Causes of overtraining

It is difficult to state (let alone investigate) what causes overtraining, as it is usually due to a combination of several factors and not just a single one. In relation to training or participating in activity, the main training factors that can lead to a state of over-training include those in table 4.11.

Table 4.11 Possible factors of overtraining

Factor	Reason
Recovery	It is common that individuals are not always given enough time for recovery between training sessions.
Frequency	Sometimes the number of training sessions per week is too high, which means that the athlete doesn't recover between sessions.
Intensity	Increasing the intensity of training sessions too quickly or by too great a jump can be detrimental.
Duration	Training sessions that are too long can cause problems as fuel storage cannot always be regenerated for the next session.
Volume	The total volume of training should only be increased by small amounts to avoid the possibility of overtraining.
Competition	It is sometimes the case that too many competitions can cause overtraining as there is psychological stress as well as physiological stress involved.

Measuring overtraining

One of the reasons why there is debate about whether or not overtraining exists is that there is no accepted method of measuring it. The other problem is that if there is a misdiagnosis of overtraining, it is possible that either the individual might push themselves too far and become ill or training might be reduced for no reason. However, even with the difficulties mentioned, there are many ways in which coaches and scientists try to measure overtraining. Some methods, for example hormonal and immune system testing, can be very expensive and only available to certain athletes.

A common method, often used if facilities and equipment are available, is a test called 'ergometry' (for measuring work rate) using, for example, a cycle ergometer with cyclists or a treadmill with runners. During this test, measures of decreases in workload, maximum heart rate and maximal blood lactate concentration are all used to try to identify overtraining.

If no appropriate equipment is available, one of the simplest ways to measure overtraining (which is easy and inexpensive) is a method known as 'mood-state' testing, with the profile of mood states (POMS) questionnaire being the most common way to do this. The POMS was originally developed in 1971 as an assessment method for people undergoing counselling or psychotherapy, but was then developed for use with people who participated in sport or exercise. As the POMS questionnaire took a relatively long time to administer (with 65 questions), a shorter one has since been developed to help assess performance and associated mood. Individuals are recommended to use the questionnaire on a daily basis to help identify any signs of overtraining. It is generally used for older children above the age of 12 but they need to have it explained to them before they use it on a regular basis. The questionnaire, which includes various statements, is normally completed on a daily basis by the individual, who rates each statement on a scale of one to five as shown in figure 4.13 so that they can keep a daily score.

Fig. 4.13 Short POMS questionnaire

Please read the statements below and give them a score of 1–5 based on the following:

1 = strongly disagree   2 = disagree   3 = neutral   4 = agree   5 = strongly agree   **Score**

- -

I slept well last night...   ......
I am looking forward to today's workout...................................   ......
I am optimistic about future performances................................   ......
I feel vigorous and energetic...   ......
I have little muscle soreness...   ......
My appetite is great..   ......

- -

TOTAL: ......

If the score is 20 or above, the individual is considered to be recovered enough to continue with the training programme that they are following. If the score is below 20, rest or an easy workout is recommended until the score rises above 20. When correctly used, the POMS scale has been shown to be effective in providing an early indication of overtraining. The coach needs to be aware, however, that the answers given are very subjective and that an individual may not be fully honest when filling out the questionnaire, especially if it might potentially cost them their place on a team.

CHAPTER FIVE
Training guidelines

Objectives

After completing this chapter the reader should be able to:

- Define the terms 'cardiovascular endurance', 'resistance training' and 'flexibility'.
- Discuss published guidelines relating to these areas of training.
- List the teaching points for a range of resistance exercises.
- List the teaching points for a range of stretching exercises.
- Explain the meaning of the terms 'static balance' and 'dynamic balance' and discuss progression methods for training these elements.
- Define the term 'speed' and discuss components related to this area of training.
- List the teaching points for a range of exercises for developing speed.
- Define the term 'agility' and discuss components related to this area of training.
- Discuss various methods of training for developing agility.
- Define the term 'power' and discuss components related to this area of training.
- List the teaching points for a range of plyometric exercises for developing power.

Introduction

When it comes to the coach trying to periodise (plan a long-term programme) from all the different components of fitness, it can be confusing as to where to start. Therefore, this chapter is concerned with training guidelines for the components of fitness that were described in chapter 4. There appear to be more published guidelines available for certain components of fitness than for others, so we will focus first on those particular components that have more sources to refer to.

Cardiovascular endurance

As described in chapter 4, cardiovascular endurance training is often just shortened to aerobic training but can refer to anaerobic-type training as well. It is often difficult for the coach to know how much cardiovascular training to prescribe for children, as the guidance from sources can be very different and often confusing. For this reason, coaches should rely only on information from credible sources (e.g. those referred to in this book) or from actual research journals.

Did you know
Professor Andy Jones, the physiologist for Paula Radcliffe, has found that beetroot juice can really help improve endurance!

There is a great deal of research which states that long-duration cardiovascular (aerobic) training is inadvisable for children, as they do not have the underpinning strength to support posture and coordination over long periods. If an exercise session is too long, children could become fatigued, which is when they are at their greatest risk of injury. The coach should, therefore, always make sure that the technique of all the players is maintained during any cardiovascular training session. If the technique of any of the players appears to become worse as the session goes on, that might be a sign that the sessions are too long and the players are fatigued. It is also quite commonly agreed that coaches should introduce short (in terms of time) bursts of high-intensity (anaerobic) training within aerobic sessions, but ensuring that there is enough time for children to recover between the bursts. It would make sense to introduce these bursts gradually and monitor how the children cope before including more of them.

Cardiovascular guidelines
As a guideline, most experts in the field agree upon an accumulation of at least 30 minutes of moderate to vigorous activity on most and preferably all days of the week

Table 5.1 Exercise guidelines for children aged 3–5 years
1 Accumulate at least 60 minutes daily of structured physical activity.
2 Engage in at least 60 minutes and up to several hours per day of unstructured physical activity and not be sedentary for more than 60 minutes at a time except when sleeping.
3 Develop competence in movement skills that are building blocks for more complex movement tasks.
4 Have indoor and outdoor areas that meet or exceed recommended safety standards for performing large-muscle activities.
5 Individuals responsible for the well-being of a preschooler should be aware of the importance of physical activity and facilitate the child's movement skills.

(the terms moderate and vigorous are subjective but the RPE scale could be used). General cardiovascular exercise guidelines for younger children (3–5 years of age) have been published by the National Association for Sport and Physical Education (NASPE) and are shown in table 5.1.

It is interesting to note that the NASPE guidelines recommend that children should not be sedentary for longer than 60-minute periods. This is obviously out of the hands of the coach and something they could only advise parents or guardians about. It is also interesting that these guidelines emphasise simple movement skills, which is supported and reiterated throughout this book. ACSM has also published guidelines, which are updated on a regular basis, in relation to children and cardiovascular exercise. In terms of age range, they are not as specific as the NASPE guidelines – the ACSM guidelines apply for all children up to the age of 16 years, although they do make specific reference to very young children. Table 5.2 gives a simplified version of the main points of the ACSM guidelines in relation to intensity, duration and frequency.

Table 5.2 ACSM cardiovascular training guidelines for children up to the age of 16 years

Intensity	Duration	Frequency
● Up to vigorous exercise ● Intermittent in nature ● For younger children, emphasis on active play rather than exercise	● 20–30 minutes ● 30–60 minutes for overweight and obese	● At least 3 days per week ● 6–7 days per week for overweight and obese

It is interesting to note, however, that ACSM recommends that to make improvements in VO_2max, children should train with heart rates of about 170–180 beats per minute, which is a heart rate range recommended by many different sources. The coach would obviously need to use heart rate monitors to be able to do this. If children do not like to train wearing heart rate monitors, the coach could get them to do one session with them on and use the RPE scale when their heart rates are in the training range; they would then be able to use the RPE in following sessions as they would know what level to work at. However, this would need to be repeated every few weeks because as children become fitter, their working RPE level changes. Check out the top tips in table 5.3 for cardiovascular training for children.

Muscular strength and endurance

The concept of resistance training is far from being a relatively recent one as it can be traced back many centuries: indeed, it has been documented that, as far back as the

---

Table 5.3 Top tips for cardiovascular training for children

1 Try to use grass or soft surfaces for activities.

2 Keep activities varied during early childhood and introduce more sports-specific ones around puberty.

3 Keep activity sessions relatively short and include bursts of vigorous intensity to see if children can cope.

4 Try not to overemphasise competition too early.

5 Use an RPE scale to monitor intensity.

6 Always have water available during all kinds of weather.

7 Monitor children at all times for fatigue in order to reduce the risk of injury.

8 Try doing occasional heart rate monitoring sessions to check the heart rate ranges.

6th century BC, progressive resistance training was practised by Milo of Crotona (a military hero and six-times Olympic champion) for the possible purpose of improving athletic ability. History suggests that Milo trained by regularly lifting a calf and, as the calf grew, the weight of the calf and hence the resistance obviously increased.

It has been said anecdotally for years that resistance training should not be done by pre-pubescent children. Current research, however, has shown that this is not really the case. There has been a great deal of research done which suggests that resistance training in children is not only safe but can also be quite effective. According to BASES, all young people should be encouraged to participate in safe and effective resistance exercise at least twice a week. To date, even though research has demonstrated that muscular strength can be increased by regular progressive resistance exercise, it is still unclear as to which resistance training programme would produce the greatest strength gains for a specific individual. As with all resistance training programmes, though, higher repetitions with low weights should be used for beginners to resistance training before progressing to heavier weights.

The problem for coaches is how much weight (or what intensity) to use when training children. Setting the intensity for resistance training can be done in several ways, with 'repetition maximum' (RM) being one of the easiest for children. Repetition maximum simply means the maximum amount of weight that can be lifted with good form for the number of repetitions chosen. For example, 6RM is the maximum amount of weight that can be lifted 6 times with good form but then causes failure on the 7th repetition.

Resistance training guidelines

As with all areas of training for children, there are many guidelines available to the coach from a number of sources. According to the Strength and Conditioning Journal, it is recommended that children do 1–3 sets of 6–15 repetitions on a variety of single- and multi-joint exercises. The guidelines from ACSM are more specific than that, however, as can be seen in table 5.4. They do not recommend an age range, but I would suggest using them for children over the age of 13–14 years.

Table 5.4 ACSM resistance training guidelines		
Intensity	**Duration**	**Frequency**
• Use weights that allow 8–15 repetitions with good form • Avoid muscular fatigue • Overload by increasing repetitions then intensity	• Perform 1 or 2 sets of 8–10 different exercises • 1–2 minutes rest between exercises • Balance major muscle groups	• 2 sessions per week • Encourage other forms of exercise

Although both sources recommend a range for the repetitions, the coach should always err on the side of caution and start those new to resistance training with the higher repetitions in the range (15 in this case). This means that coaches should help children to find the weights, for each exercise that has been chosen, with which they can do 15 repetitions but not 16. After a few weeks, however, children will become stronger, which means that they will naturally be able to do more than 15 repetitions with the weight that was first selected. Therefore, they are ready to progress so the coach should allow more weight to be selected. Be aware, though, that progression should be slow, so only small amounts of weight should be added at this stage.

As well as information relating to sets, repetitions, rest and so on, there are many guidelines, from a variety of sources, relating to general resistance training. These guidelines tend to be similar, however, regardless of the source. There are many training methods that can be used to develop muscular strength or endurance (*see* chapter 4 for a definition). These methods include resistance training using machines and free weights, body-weight training and resistance training bands.

Body-weight exercises

The full range of resistance training exercises available is beyond the scope of this book but figures 5.1 to 5.10 show a selection of body-weight exercises that can be used: these would be an appropriate starting point for many children who are not familiar with or experienced in resistance training.

BOX PRESS-UP
Main muscles used: pectorals, triceps

Technique:

1 Make a box shape with the body as in figure 5.1(a) with the arms out straight and hands flat on the floor directly under the shoulders
2 Under control, lower the body until the chin is a few centimetres off the floor as in figure 5.1(b) (this is called the mid-position)
3 Return to the start position

Awareness:
Keep the head looking down at the floor so it doesn't put undue stress on the neck.

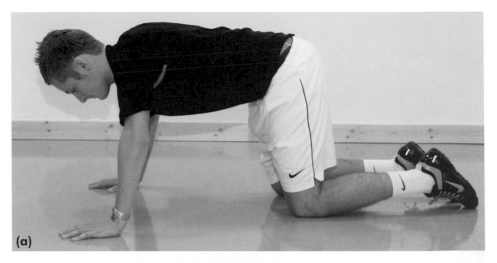

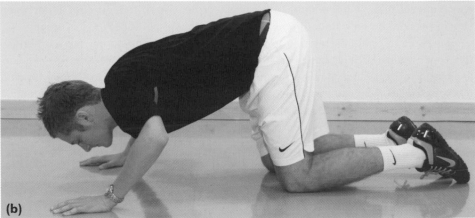

Fig. 5.1 Box press-up (a) Start position (b) Mid-position

THREE-QUARTER PRESS-UP
Main muscles used: pectorals, triceps

Technique:

1 Start with the knees on the floor as in figure 5.2(a) with the arms out straight and hands flat on the floor – a straight line should be made through the body from the knees upward
2 Under control, lower the body until the chest is a few centimetres off the floor as in figure 5.2(b) (this is called the mid-position)
3 Return to the start position

Awareness:
Use a mat below the knees as this press-up can be uncomfortable.

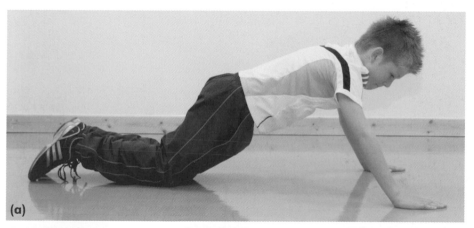

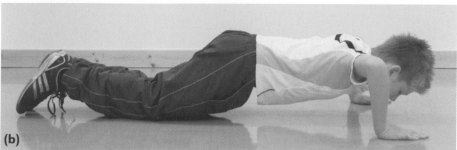

Fig. 5.2 Three-quarter press-up (a) Start position (b) Mid-position

FULL PRESS-UP
Main muscles used: pectorals, triceps

Technique:

1 A straight line through the body should be made as in figure 5.3(a) with the arms out straight and hands flat on the floor
2 Under control, lower the body until the chest is a few centimetres off the floor as in figure 5.3(b) (this is called the mid-position)
3 Return to the start position

Awareness:
Start children with the box or three-quarter press-up to make sure they are strong enough to do a full press-up.

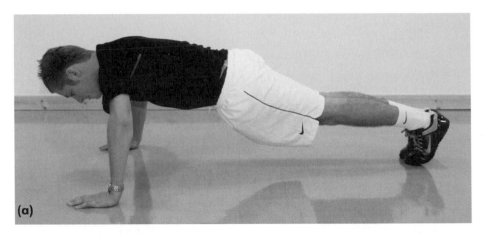

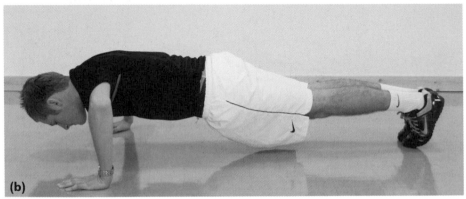

Fig. 5.3 Full press-up (a) Start position (b) Mid-position

SQUAT
Main muscles used: quadriceps, hamstrings, glutes

Technique:

1 Stand upright with the feet shoulder-width apart as in figure 5.4(a)
2 Slowly descend as if trying to sit on a chair – each individual should squat as far as they are comfortable (mid-position as in fig. 5.4(b))
3 Return to the start position

Awareness:
If children start to raise the heels off the floor this may be an indication that the calf muscles are tight – children should be encouraged to squat as far as they can to maintain their range of motion and to help build strength in this position.

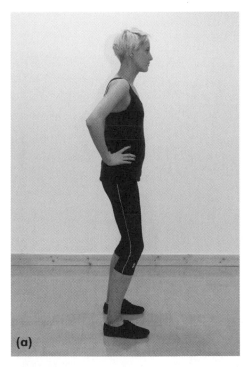
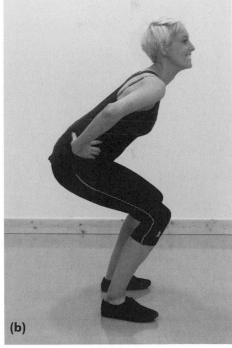

Fig. 5.4 Squat (a) Start position (b) Mid-position

WALL SQUAT
Main muscles used: quadriceps, hamstrings, glutes

Technique:

1 A flat wall is needed for this exercise
2 Stand against the wall with the feet about 30–45 centimetres away from the wall as in figure 5.5(a) – the feet should be shoulder-width apart
3 Slide down the wall until the thighs are parallel with the floor as in figure 5.5(b)
4 Hold this position for a few seconds then return to the start position

Awareness:
This exercise is usually done as a static exercise – in other words, hold the mid-position for a few seconds without moving before returning to the start position.

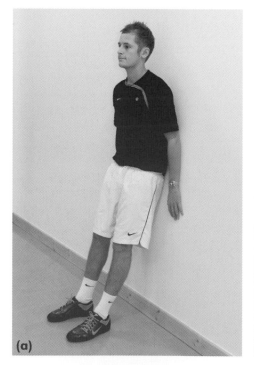 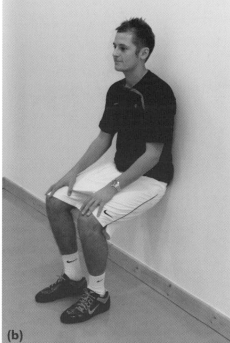

(a)   (b)

Fig. 5.5 Wall squat (a) Start position (b) Mid-position

FRONT LUNGE

Main muscles used: quadriceps, hamstrings, glutes, calves

Technique:

1 Start from an upright position with the feet slightly apart as in figure 5.6(a)
2 Take a small step forwards and lower the body down until the front thigh is parallel to the ground as in figure 5.6(b)
3 Return to the start position and repeat with the other leg

Awareness:
- Keep the upper body upright throughout the exercise
- Try to avoid the front knee going beyond the line of the toes

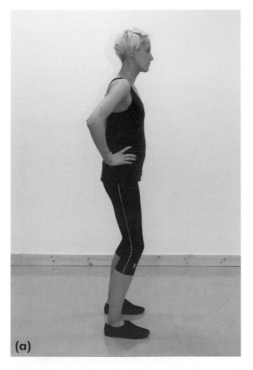
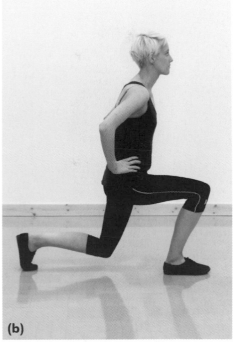

Fig. 5.7 Front lunge (a) Start position (b) Mid-position

ANGLE LUNGE

Main muscles used: quadriceps, hamstrings, glutes, calves, abductors, adductors

Technique:

1 Start from an upright position with the feet slightly apart as in figure 5.7(a)
2 Take a small step forwards at an angle of about 45 degrees and lower the body down until the front thigh is parallel to the ground as in figure 5.7(b)
3 Return to the start position and repeat with the other leg

Awareness:
- Keep the upper body upright throughout the exercise
- Vary the angle of the lunges so that children experience lunging through the full 360 degrees around the body

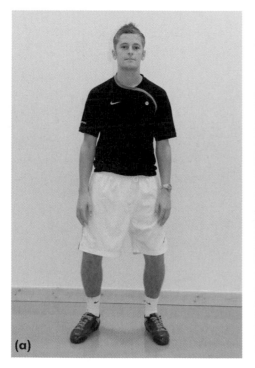 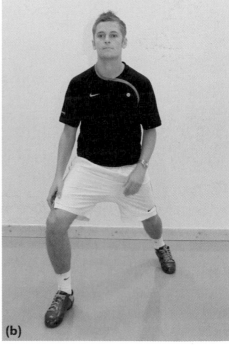

Fig. 5.7 Angle lunge (a) Start position (b) Mid-position

DIP

Main muscles used: triceps

Technique:

1 A chair or bench is needed for this exercise
2 Start with the hands on the edge of the chair or bench – the arms should be at full extension and the legs out straight as in figure 5.8(a)
3 Slowly lower the body down until the upper arms are just above parallel to the floor as in figure 5.8(b)
4 Return to the start position

Awareness:
● Do not do this exercise if children have or are recovering from any shoulder injury
● Limit the range of the descent as described in the technique

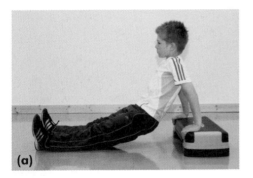 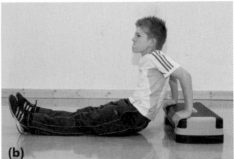

Fig. 5.8 Dip (a) Start position (b) Mid-position

STEP-UP

Main muscles used: quadriceps, hamstrings, glutes, calves

Technique:

1 A bench or platform is needed for this exercise
2 Start about 30 centimetres from the bench in an upright position as in figure 5.9(a)
3 Place one foot on the bench and step up as in figure 5.9(b)
4 Return to the start position by stepping down under control

Awareness:

● Start with a bench height that is about 15 centimetres below the knee of the performer
● Always step down under control onto the ball of the foot
● Ensure the leg that is used to step up and down is alternated

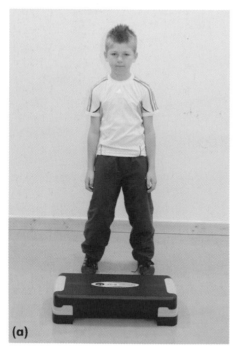 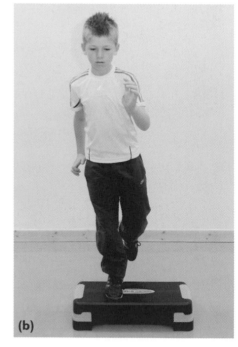

(a) (b)

Fig. 5.9 Step-up (a) Start position (b) Mid-position

BACK EXTENSION
Main muscles used: erector spinae

Technique:

1 Lie face down on the floor as in figure 5.10(a) and place the hands to the sides of the head
2 Raise the upper body a few centimetres off the floor as in figure 5.10(b)
3 Lower the body back down to the start position

Awareness:
- Do not be tempted to put the hands behind the head
- Encourage children not to support the body with the hands
- Limit the range of motion to only a few centimetres

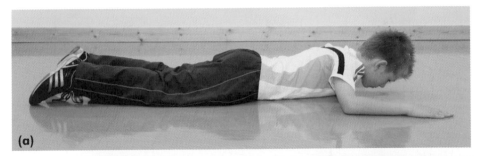

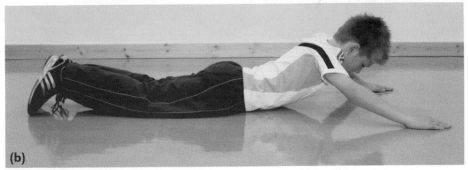

Fig. 5.10 Back extension (a) Start position (b) Mid-position

Order of resistance training

The coach should be aware that there are many combinations of possible resistance exercises that could be chosen. However, there seems to be more and more research that recommends general exercises such as lunging, bending, pushing and pulling in order to develop these motor skills and movement coordination, as opposed to isolated machine-based training such as leg-curls and chest presses. If the coach is just prescribing a whole-body resistance training programme, there is a general rule that could be followed: train large muscles before small ones. For instance, table 5.5 shows a typical whole-body workout that could be done in the same session.

Table 5.5 Typical whole-body resistance workout (in order)	
Muscle	**Exercise**
Chest (pecs)	Pec dec or chest press or press-up or chest fly
Back (lats)	Lat pull-down or pull-up or single-arm row
Shoulders (delts)	Shoulder press or lateral raise
Arms (biceps)	Biceps curl
Arms (triceps)	Triceps push-down or dip
Buttocks (glutes)	Squat
Front thigh (quads)	Leg extension or squat
Back thigh (hams)	Leg curl or squat
Back shin (calves)	Calf raise or lunge

The session in table 5.5 could be done in the order it appears or the legs could be done before the upper body. This might depend on whether or not the player had just finished a cardio session in which the legs were fatigued. If this was the case, the coach could also decide to do the upper body on one day and the legs on another. Finding the ideal method for players is very much a trial and error affair in which dialogue between the player and the coach is essential to monitor the progress of the training and to adjust it if necessary. Table 5.6 gives a list of top tips for resistance training for children.

Table 5.6 Top tips for resistance training for children

1 Supervise all resistance training activities at all times.

2 Advise individuals to learn technique before trying to increase strength.

3 Start with body-weight exercises before moving on to any type of weight exercise.

4 Encourage children to always perform a full range of motion regardless of the exercise.

5 Be in control of the movement.

6 Avoid ballistic movements.

7 Make sure all major muscle groups in the body are trained each week.

8 Focus on general motor skill movements as opposed to isolated muscle exercises.

Flexibility

When a stretch is performed and held for a period of time, it is usually referred to as a 'static' stretch. If a partner assists or another group of muscles (by the person stretching) is used in this process, it is called an 'active' stretch. If there is no assistance in the stretch, it is said to be a 'passive' stretch. Static stretching is associated with 'end range of motion' and physiological adaptation of tissues so it is recommended to perform this type of stretch after exercise.

If a stretch is done in motion it is referred to as a 'dynamic' stretch. Stretches of this type are normally associated with warm-ups as they provide a rehearsal almost of the activities to follow. It is interesting that children are naturally quite flexible, yet they are constantly being encouraged to perform long-duration static stretching (especially in gymnastic-type events). A certain amount of flexibility is required for most sports, with some sports requiring more than others (refer to the flexibility task in chapter 4), but the majority of children will already have the necessary flexibility.

Flexibility guidelines

Generally speaking, flexibility is maintained until the age of about 10–12 years, at which point children will slowly begin to lose flexibility, particularly around the hips and shoulders. For this reason, dynamic exercises or activities that encourage active range of motion, such as squats, lunges, high knees and skips, should be enough to maintain flexibility for younger children. There are published guidelines, however, that relate to children. For example, from the age of 12 years onwards the ACSM guidelines for flexibility shown in table 5.7 could be used in most cases.

Table 5.7 ACSM guidelines for flexibility		
Intensity	**Duration**	**Frequency**
● To the end range of motion ● A point of tightness without pain	● Hold for 15–30 seconds ● Repeat 2–4 times for each stretch	● A minimum of 2–3 sessions per week ● Ideally 5–7 sessions per week

The ACSM guidelines appear only to refer to static-type stretches and do not give any indication of when to perform them. For the purpose of this book, we shall assume that static stretches will be done at the end of a session following the cool-down, and dynamic-type stretches will be done at the start of a session either following or as part of the warm-up.

Dynamic stretches

There are many dynamic-type stretches that can be done prior to activity sessions. Coaches can simply devise their own stretches that mimic the movements of a particular sport or event, or they can assign the same movements, at a slower speed and lower intensity, that will be done later in the main activity session. Figures 5.11 to 5.18 give a description of just some of the dynamic stretches that can be done.

BALLS OF FEET

Main muscles stretched: tibialis anterior (front of the shin)

Technique:

1 Rise up onto the ball of one foot as in figure 5.11(a) and then lower under control
2 Do this on the other leg and repeat several times

Progression:

- Walking heel raise – while walking forwards rise up onto the ball of each foot
- Jogging slowly, point the toes of the foot off the ground at the floor in front as in figure 5.11(b)

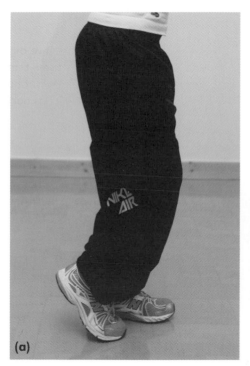
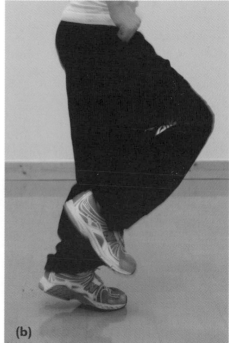

Fig. 5.11 Balls of feet (a) On the spot (b) Jogging

GOOSE STEP
Main muscles stretched: hamstrings (back of the thigh), calf (back of the shin)

Technique:

1 From a standing position lift one knee and then straighten out the leg at about a 45-degree angle with the toes pulled back as in figure 5.12
2 Repeat with the other leg

Progression:
- While walking, pull the toes back on the leading leg, while at the same time extending the heel and maintaining a straight leg
- This can be done at a jogging pace but it becomes more like skipping

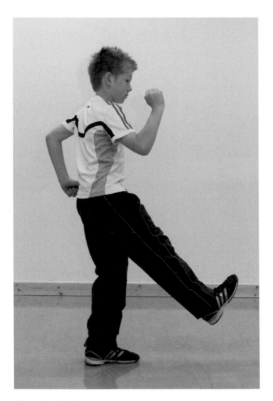

Fig. 5.12 Goose step

KNEE HUG

Main muscles stretched: gluteus muscles (buttocks)

Technique:

1 From a standing position lift one knee and pull it towards the chest as in figure 5.13
2 Repeat with the other leg

Progression:
- While walking, pull the knee to the chest, keeping an upright posture
- Try this while jogging or skipping

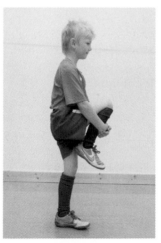

Fig. 5.13 Knee hug

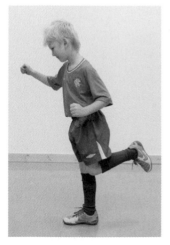

Fig. 5.14 Leg curl

LEG CURL

Main muscles stretched: hamstrings (back of thigh)

Technique:

1 From a standing position lift one foot off the floor and bring it towards the buttocks, keeping the thigh as vertical as possible as in figure 5.14
2 Repeat with the other leg

Progression:
- While walking, bring the heel towards the buttocks, keeping an upright posture and the thigh vertical
- Try this while jogging or skipping

BOWLING

Main muscles stretched: hamstrings (back of thigh)

Technique:

1 From a standing position put one leg about 30 centimetres out in front of the other
2 In a smooth action, bend the back leg at the knee as if trying to sit down
3 Keep the body upright as you are doing this and pull the toes of the front leg towards you as in figure 5.15
4 Go back to the start and do the other leg

Progression:
- Do this while walking, almost mimicking a crown green bowling action
- This is not suitable for a jogging pace

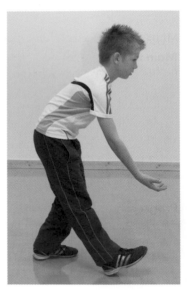

Fig. 5.15 Bowling

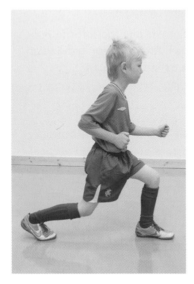

Fig. 5.16 Lunge

LUNGE

Main muscles stretched: hip flexors (front of hip)

Technique:

1 From a standing position take a large step forwards (called a split stance)
2 Bend the front leg at the knee so that the back leg is straight and the body lowers as in figure 5.16
3 Come back to a standing position and change legs

Progression:
- Do this while walking and keeping an upright posture
- This is not suitable for a jogging pace

HURDLE

Main muscles stretched: hip adductors and abductors (inside and outside of the upper thigh)

Technique:

1 From a standing position mimic the trailing leg of a hurdler going over a hurdle as in figure 5.17
2 Bring the leg back to the start and change legs

Progression:
- Do this while walking and keeping an upright posture
- Try this at jogging pace but only raise each leg after every 3 or 4 paces

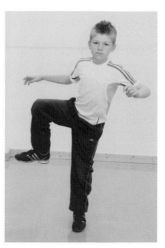

Fig. 5.17 Hurdle

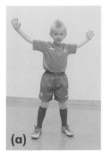

(a)

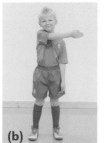

(b)

ARM SWING

Main muscles stretched: chest and back muscle groups

Technique:

1 In a standing position swing the arms (in a controlled way) out and away from the body at an angle as in figure 5.18(a) and then across the body as in figure 5.18(b)
2 Repeat, swinging the arms out and away from the body at different angles each time

Progression:
- Do this while walking and keeping an upright posture
- Try this at jogging pace but only do an arm swing after every 3 or 4 paces

Fig. 5.18 Arm swing
(a) Swing out (b) Swing across

Static stretches

Static stretches are usually limited to main muscle groups and are usually performed at the end of the session. Figures 5.19 to 5.27 show how to carry out common static stretches for the main muscle groups.

CHEST STRETCH

Main muscles stretched: pectorals (chest), biceps (front of upper arm), anterior deltoid (front of shoulder)

Technique:

1 Stand with the feet hip-width apart and clasp the hands behind the back as in the start position in figure 5.19(a)
2 From this position, straighten and raise the arms until tension is felt as in the end position in figure 5.19(b)

Awareness:
- Maintain good posture throughout the stretch and try not to lean forwards
- Stretch may be done in a standing or seated position
- Some children might be very flexible and not feel this stretch, so they should just raise their arms as far as they can

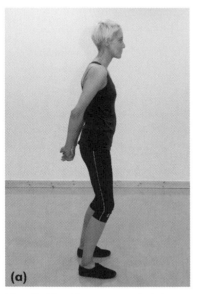 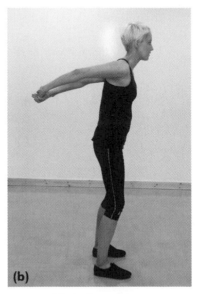

(a) (b)

Fig. 5.19 Chest stretch (a) Start position (b) End position

BACK STRETCH

Main muscles stretched: trapezius (middle of back), latissimus dorsi (lower and middle back), posterior deltoid (back of shoulder), biceps (front of upper arm)

Technique:

1 Stand with the feet hip-width apart and clasp the hands in front of the body
2 Straighten the arms out from the body while trying to separate the shoulder blades by pushing the shoulders forwards as in figure 5.20

Awareness:

- Stretch may be done with a slight lean forwards and in a standing or seated position
- The arms should be approximately parallel to the floor

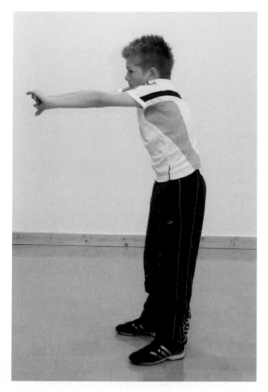

Fig. 5.20 Back stretch

BACK OF ARM STRETCH
Main muscles stretched: triceps (back of upper arm)

Technique:

1 Stand with the feet hip-width apart and raise one arm above the head with the palm facing backwards as in the start position in figure 5.21(a)

2 From this position, try to touch the shoulder blade on the same side of the body as in the end position in figure 5.21(b)

Awareness:
- Maintain good posture throughout the stretch and keep the upper arm vertical
- Stretch may be done in a standing or seated position
- If no stretch is felt, use the opposite hand to push back at the elbow

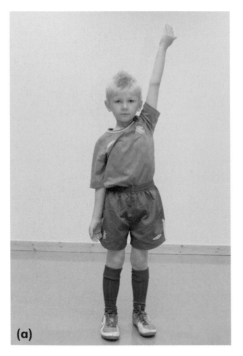 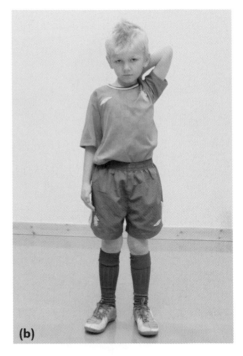

(a)   (b)

Fig. 5.21 Back of arm stretch (a) Start position (b) End position

HIP STRETCH
Main muscles stretched: hip flexors (front of the hip)

Technique:

1 Adopt a lunge position as in figure 5.22(a)
2 From this position lower the hip forwards slightly and down – keep the body upright as you are doing this
3 Lower until tension is felt in the hip as in the end position in figure 5.22(b)

Awareness:
- Maintain an upright posture throughout the stretch
- Keep the front foot flat on the floor and the back leg on the ball of the foot

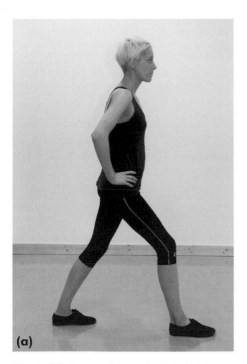
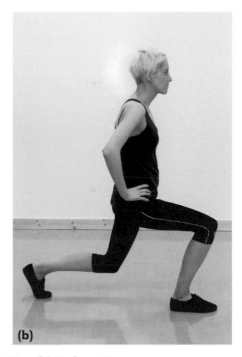

(a)   (b)

Fig. 5.22 Front of hip stretch (a) Start position (b) End position

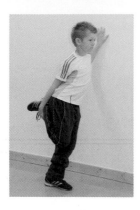

Fig. 5.23 Front of thigh stretch

FRONT OF THIGH STRETCH

Main muscles stretched: quadriceps (front of the thigh)

Technique:

1 Stand upright with both feet close together
2 Lift one foot off the ground so that the heel comes towards the buttocks
3 Take hold of the front of the raised foot and squeeze the heel further towards the buttocks keeping the legs close together as in figure 5.23

Awareness:

● Maintain an upright posture throughout the stretch
● The supporting leg can be slightly bent
● Keep the upper part of the stretched leg vertical and do not let it move forwards

BACK OF THIGH STRETCH

Main muscles stretched: hamstrings (back of the thigh)

Technique:

1 From a standing position put one leg about 30 centimetres out in front of the other
2 Bend the back leg at the knee as if trying to sit down – keep the body upright as you are doing this and pull the toes of the front leg towards you as in figure 5.24
3 Lower the body until tension is felt in the back of the thigh

Awareness:

● Keep an upright posture throughout the stretch
● You can support yourself by putting your hands on the knee of the bent leg

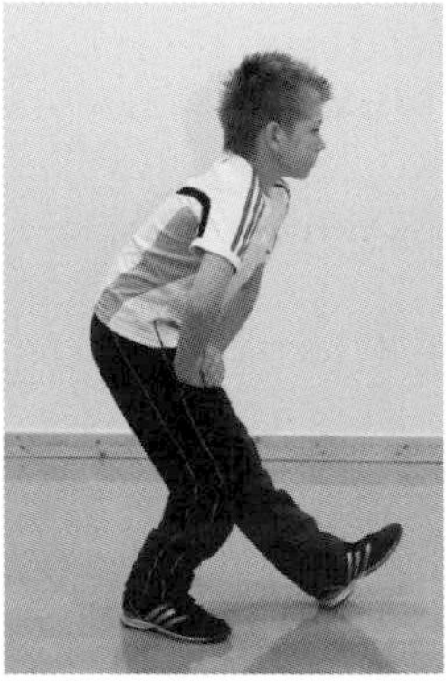

Fig. 5.24 Back of thigh stretch

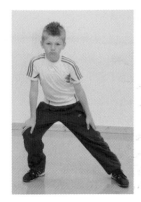

Fig. 5.25 Inside of thigh stretch

INSIDE OF THIGH STRETCH

Main muscles stretched: hip adductors (inside of the upper thigh)

Technique:

1 Stand upright with the legs apart (just slightly more than shoulder-width)
2 Bend the knee of one leg so that it goes forwards and at the same time lean to the side (of the bent knee) and keep the opposite leg straight as in figure 5.25
3 Lower the body until tension is felt in the inside of the thigh of the straight leg

Awareness:
- Maintain an upright posture throughout the stretch
- Try to lean only to the side and not forwards or backwards

OUTSIDE OF THIGH STRETCH

Main muscles stretched: hip abductors (outside of the upper thigh)

Technique:

1 Take a seated position with the legs together out straight
2 Bring one knee towards you and place the foot over the straight leg as in the start position in figure 5.26(a)
3 Sit upright and hug the bent knee while trying to pull it towards the opposite shoulder as in the end position in figure 5.26(b)

Awareness:
- Maintain an upright posture throughout the stretch
- Try not to twist the upper body
- Keep the non-stretching leg out straight

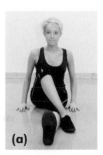

(a)

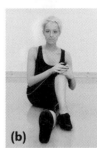

(b)

Fig. 5.26 Outside of thigh stretch (a) Start position (b) End position

BACK OF LOWER LEG STRETCH
Main muscles stretched: calf (back of the lower leg)

Technique:

1 From a standing position take a step backwards as in the start position in figure 5.27(a)
2 Bend the front knee and lean forwards keeping the back leg straight and foot flat on the floor as in the end position in figure 5.27(b)

Awareness:
- Maintain an upright posture throughout the stretch
- Keep the back leg straight with the foot flat on the floor at all times
- Try not to let the front knee go in front of the toe line

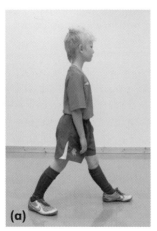 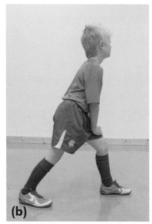

Fig. 5.27 Back of lower leg stretch (a) Start position (b) End position

It is difficult trying to introduce a new stretching routine to adults, but for children it should be reasonably easy to develop routines as early as possible. Children should then get into the habit of doing dynamic-type stretches before main sessions and static-type stretches after sessions. Once they do, it is likely they will continue even when not under the direct supervision of the coach as is often the case when players do their own training.

Professional teams are a good role model but sometimes it is not always evident as they tend to stretch dynamically a little while before the game starts, and then come back out onto the pitch to do their cool-down and stretches a short time after the game ends. Get children to watch out for this. For instance, after a football game, you can often see players back out on the pitch behind the panel in the studio who are doing after-match assessments. Table 5.8 gives a list of top tips for stretching.

Table 5.8 Top tips for stretching
1 Never stretch when cold.
2 Use dynamic-type stretches before a main activity.
3 Use static-type stretches after activities.
4 Try not to develop too much flexibility unless it is absolutely necessary for the demands of the sport.
5 Never stretch to the point of pain.
6 Develop stretching habits at an early age.

Balance

Even though balance is considered to be an essential component of any sport, event or activity, there is little in the way of guidelines relating to this component of fitness. It is generally agreed, however, that static balance (*see* chapter 4) should be developed before dynamic balance. In scientific terms, static balance relates to keeping the centre of mass within the base of support. In simple terms this means trying not to fall over.

Definition
The 'base of support' just means the parts of the body in contact with the floor that are keeping the balance.

Static balance

In order to develop balance skills, the demand on the body to balance must be increased. Static balance can be developed in various ways, such as by changing the base of support. If the base of support is made smaller, by bringing the feet closer together for example, then the demand for balance will be greater. As balance relies heavily on visual input (sight), if this is taken away by closing the eyes, the demand to use other senses for balance will be increased. Adding another skill, such as catching while trying to balance, would not only take the attention away from balancing to concentrate on catching, but also increase the demand on the vestibular system (*see* chapter 4) to maintain balance. Table 5.9 shows how static balance skills could be progressed to increase the balance demand on the various systems in the body.

Table 5.9 Progression of static balance

Skill	Progression	Demand
Children stand, looking forwards, with feet hip-width apart and arms outstretched. Try this again but with the feet closer together.	• Hold up different cards (numbered or coloured) and get children to shout out the number or colour as quickly as possible. • In pairs, one child throws a ball to the child balancing. • Get children to close their eyes and remain as still as possible. • With the eyes closed, get children to pass a ball around a circle.	• Increases demand on proprioception (see page 83) and the vestibular system (see page 84) as attention is deflected. • As above but attention is deflected even more. • Increases demand on proprioception and vestibular system as visual input is reduced. • Increases demand on proprioception and vestibular system as movement is added.
Children stand, looking forwards, with feet close together and arms outstretched.	• Get children to lift one foot a few centimetres off the floor and hold. • Introduce catching skill while holding one foot off the floor. • With the foot off the floor, try closing the eyes.	• Increases demand mainly on proprioception. • Increases demand on vestibular system and proprioception. • Heavy demand on vestibular and proprioceptive systems.

Coaches might be familiar with balance training that involves the use of equipment such as wobble-boards (these are inflatable rubber discs about 30 centimetres in diameter). As there is some evidence to show that the risk of injury might be increased by the use of such equipment (mainly to the ankle joints, as it is thought that children are not strong enough to support the balance demands of the excessive ankle movement), I would prefer to err on the side of caution and recommend that balance training should be done without such equipment.

Dynamic balance

Dynamic balance is also a component that needs to be developed in childhood as most sports and events require a high degree of this component of fitness. For instance, dynamic balance is needed when landing on one foot or both feet and coming to a stop, or it may be required when landing on one foot or both feet but then carrying on the movement, as in an agility-type skill. Table 5.10 shows how typical dynamic balance skills can be progressed in terms of the balance demand of the various body systems.

Table 5.10 Typical dynamic balance skills and progressions

Skill	Progression
As in a broad jump, children take off and land on both feet under control.	• Increase the length of the jump. • Increase the height of the jump. • Jump out at a slight angle, i.e. not straight. • Land with feet together, feet apart, feet in split stance etc. • Try to land on targets.
As above but land on one foot.	• Increase the length of the jump. • Increase the height of the jump. • Jump out at a slight angle, i.e. not straight. • Try to land on targets.
Land on both feet, as in a broad jump, but then take off again.	• Start with short jumps then increase the length. • Start with jumps in a straight line then change direction of jump. • Just do one extra take-off. • Try multiple take-offs. • Try adding an object, such as a hurdle, to jump over.
As above but on one foot.	• As above but try taking off on one foot and landing on the other, and then taking off and landing on the same foot (hopping).

As you can see in table 5.10, there are many dynamic balance exercises available but the coach must be aware that these movements are typical of the movements carried out in sport. For this reason, they should be careful and try not to repeat too often these movements in training sessions during weeks when there are game situations so as not to overload the players, as the demands placed on the joints of young players doing these types of exercise are quite high.

Speed

As mentioned in chapter 4, speed may be thought of in two ways: the speed of body movements such as punching or kicking and the speed of the whole body in any direction along the ground. For the purpose of this chapter we will focus on the latter.

As with agility, speed along the ground requires many abilities of the individual such as balance, strength and efficiency of movement. Another term for efficiency of movement is 'movement mechanics', and this is something that coaches often try to work on in training. Teaching the mechanics of movement is usually based on observation rather than on initial instruction. Although performers need to be guided through the initial elements of how to move well, much of their learning happens gradually, as information is 'drip fed'.

The 'little and often' approach to mechanics teaching can be used effectively by the reinforcement of simple instructions during an activity session. The teaching and development of good movement mechanics does not have to be a complicated process. The principles are simple and remain the same for the vast majority of movements. For example, table 5.11 describes, in relation to body parts, just some of the teaching points that can be used to help improve the efficiency of the performer.

Table 5.11 Teaching points for movement mechanics

Body part	Description	Teaching point
Elbows	Elbows at roughly 90 degrees will decrease the amount of fluctuation of the centre of gravity.	'Pocket to mouth'
Core	An upright, stable posture is efficient with respect to the transfer of power through the body.	'Stand tall'
Feet	When running, the ball of the foot should make contact with the floor as opposed to the heel or the toes.	'Light feet'
Knees	The optimum height of the knee for sprinters is about 70 degrees. Any higher than this is classed as wasted movement, as it occurs in a vertical direction. Hurdles are a useful tool for emphasising the knee drive by encouraging the runner to skim the top of the hurdle when running.	'Skim the hurdles'

Generally speaking, training methods for speed focus on increasing the stride frequency or improving the stride length of the runner (*see* chapter 4 for definitions). Downhill running and resisted training are methods normally used for this but guidelines for children are very vague. Resisted running (usually by towing weights on a sled) is commonly used in a variety of sports as a means for developing speed; however, research as to its effectiveness for adults, let alone children, is limited. Typically, track sprinters rarely tow more than 5.0–7.5% of their body weight during training, while in sports such as rugby, players rarely exceed 20% of their body weight (there are exceptions). It has been suggested that using weights in excess of this would alter the running technique (usually by decreasing the stride length and forward lean) and possibly impair its efficiency.

Speed drills

Speed drills are often performed in order to help develop 'correct' techniques and at much slower speeds than sprinting. As this is the case, they are considered to be useful as part of a warm-up prior to a main training session or event. Plyometric exercises are also used to develop speed and will be covered later in this chapter.

It is generally thought to be more difficult to increase the stride frequency than the length of stride. There are many types of exercise (drill) that are used by sprint coaches to develop speed: usually a combination of them all is used as it is difficult to know which one is the best. Figures 5.28 to 5.31 show some typical sprinting drills that are commonly practised by children, often above the age of 12 years, involved in specific sports training.

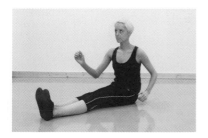

ARM-SWING DRILL

Correct arm swing during sprinting helps to decrease rotational forces within the body that can slow it down. For instance, when one leg is extended backwards it can create a turning force within the body. If the opposite arm is moved forwards it can help to counteract that turning force.

Fig. 5.28 Seated arm-swing drill

Technique:

1 The arms (bent at about 90 degrees) should be driven backwards from the shoulder when sprinting and the hand should travel from hip level to shoulder level
2 These arm-swing drills can be performed from a sitting position as in figure 5.28, progressing to doing them while walking or jogging

ANKLING DRILL

This is the term used for drills that consist of lifting one foot off the floor and placing it down correctly to try to encourage quick floor contact.

Technique:

1 The foot should look like it is trying to 'paw' the ground, only making contact with the forefoot (ball of the foot) as in figure 5.29
2 Running on the toes or from heel to toe when sprinting should be discouraged
3 This technique may take some practice before it feels right and cues such as 'toes up' and 'quick feet' can be used when performing these drills.

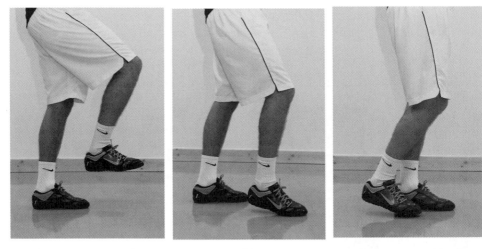

Fig. 5.29 Ankling drill: (a) Start position (b) Initial floor contact (c) Pawing the floor

HEEL-KICK (OR BUTT-KICK) DRILL

When the heel is lifted towards the buttocks (hence the alternative name 'butt-kick'), it means that the length of the leg is shorter and closer to the point of rotation (at the hip). This means that the leg can then move forwards more quickly. Drills should begin at walking pace and emphasis should be placed on one leg before progressing to using both legs or to speeding up the kick.

Technique:

1 The heel should be brought towards the buttocks as quickly as possible, followed by quickly raising and then lowering the knee as in figure 5.30
2 The individual should be encouraged not to lose the dorsiflexed (toe-up) position
3 This should look like a cycling motion

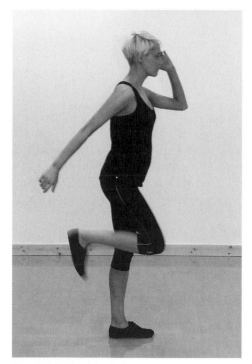

Fig. 5.30 Heel-kick (or butt-kick) drill

KNEE-LIFT DRILL

These types of drill help to teach correct knee action and foot positioning.

Technique:

1 The thigh should be lifted quickly until it is parallel to the ground with the foot dorsi-flexed (toes-up) as in figure 5.31

2 The foot should then come down and make contact with the ground just in front of the hips

3 These drills should be practised at walking pace to start with, using only one leg and then progressed to include arm action and using both legs

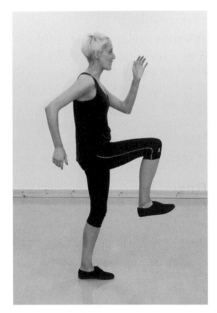

Fig. 5.31 Knee-lift drill

Agility

In relation to many sporting events, change of direction training is essential. Many sports often include repeated short sprinting with changes of direction at sprinting speeds. Coaches should be aware, however, that there is little relationship between straight sprinting ability and the ability to perform complex tasks such as dribbling a ball. In other words, a fast sprinter doesn't make a good footballer, for instance. For this reason, it is recommended that training should mimic the sporting situation as closely as possible.

'Agility drills' are just exercises involving acceleration, a change of direction at speed, and deceleration that mimic movements within a sport or event. Because of the complex nature of movements classified as 'agility', the coach should make sure that players have progressed from more simple movements and have the balance, strength and power to cope with this type of training. There are actual tests that can be done to measure agility. The coach should also take into consideration whether or not the agility drill needs to be programmed or random. For instance, the drill might just involve a simple set-up where the player has to perform a set routine when they are ready to go. On the other hand, the drill might be more complex involving anticipation of movement and identification of triggers, such as a gap in the opponent's defence. Including within agility drills a more complex reaction, such as the use of different coloured markers or varied verbal instructions (e.g. cues such as 'run to blue cone, then red, then back to centre'), will make the drills more appropriate to sporting situations. Figure 5.32 gives an example of such an agility drill.

Power

This term 'power' should really be 'muscular power', as it is related to the strength of a muscle and the speed at which it can contract. There are only a few sports in which maximal strength is required, so power is considered to be a more important component of fitness for most sports and activities. It is generally thought that heavy strength training may contribute slightly to explosive power movements; training that uses lighter resistances, however, may contribute more. Power training is often used by coaches to improve sprinting and is therefore an important component that needs to be developed in sports or events where sprinting is required.

Resistance training and power

One way to improve power in adults is by increasing the size of the muscle (called hypertrophy); coaches should be aware that for younger children, however, this type of training is not really advocated. With adults, first increasing the size of the muscles is an often-used approach to increase the force of the muscles: they can then focus on increasing the speed of the muscular contraction. Other coaches use an approach whereby they set training programmes that have a period with relatively heavy loads (over 80% of maximum), followed by a period using fairly light loads (30–50% of maximum). It is generally agreed that this type of training will increase power without gaining muscle size (this is called increasing the 'power-to-weight ratio'), but it is recommended that an individual should have a good strength base before undertaking such training.

Plyometric training

Training for children is different as their muscles are developing and growing, and so the coach needs to limit the type of power training that they do. The reason for this is that in many cases they will be doing power training without even being aware of it. For instance, one of the most common methods of training to develop power is known as 'plyometric' training, derived from Greek meaning 'changing length'. A common definition of the word 'plyometric' is 'rapid eccentric loading followed by a brief isometric phase and explosive rebound using stored elastic energy and powerful concentric contractions'. What this means in simple terms is any fast movement with rebound, for example where the foot hits the floor and takes off again in running and jumping. It is obvious, therefore, that playing sport or doing many activities can be classed as plyometric and would have the same benefits.

Plyometric guidelines

With regard to guidelines for training, a minimum age of 16 is recommended by several authors as a younger individual may not have the bone maturation to cope with the strenuous loads that this type of training places on joints. However, ACSM does not state a particular age range guideline but advises that, to minimise the likelihood of injury, participants must be closely supervised and learn the correct technique, and the training intensity and volume must not exceed the abilities of the participants.

For pre-pubertal and early pubertal children, few training studies have been undertaken in relation to plyometric training, although some have demonstrated that maximal cycling power, countermovement jumping, squat jumping, multiple bounding, repeated rebound jumping for 15 seconds and 20-metre sprinting all improved significantly following a plyometric training programme. It is recommended by many sources that a good strength base is a requirement for plyometric training due to the intense nature of the exercises and the increased risk of injury. Strength ratios of 1.5 to 2.5 times body weight for 1RM squats (lower-body plyometrics) and 1.0 to 1.5 times body weight for bench press (upper-body plyometrics) are commonly recommended. Other recommendations include the ability to perform five consecutive clap push-ups. If an individual does not posses the strength capability for either lower- or upper-body strength recommendations then it is suggested that plyometric exercises should be delayed until they do.

With beginners to this type of training it is important to focus on correct technique prior to performing any loaded or intense exercises. It is also recommended to start with soft ground outdoors before progression to harder surfaces. Figures 5.33 to 5.40 show some common plyometric exercises that can be incorporated into a training programme. The exercises are split into two groups, lower- and upper-body. The exercises chosen will be dependent on the requirements of the sport or event but each group is arranged in order of increasing difficulty: those new to plyometric training should start with the easiest exercises before progressing to the harder ones.

Lower-body plyometric exercises

TUCK JUMP

Technique:

1 Stand with the feet hip-width apart
2 Jump up off both feet and bring the knees to the chest (fig. 5.32)
3 Land on the balls of the feet and immediately jump up again
4 Try to keep the contact time with the floor as short as possible
5 If the jump is done correctly the performer will land back on the take-off spot

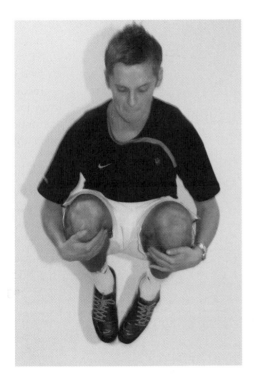

Fig. 5.32 Tuck jump

BROAD JUMP

Technique:

1 Stand with the feet hip-width apart
2 Squat down (slight forward lean), with the arms straight and back
3 Jump off both feet in a forward direction to get as far as possible (fig. 5.33(a))
4 Swing the arms through while doing this
5 Land on the balls of the feet and maintain balance (fig. 5.33(b))

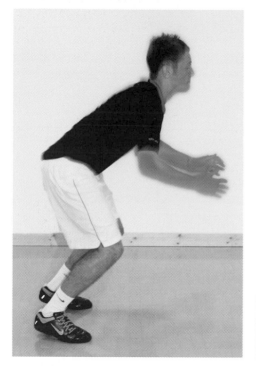
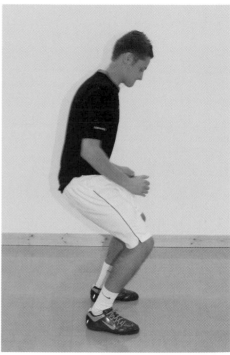

Fig. 5.33 Broad jump (a) Take-off (b) Landing

BUNNY HOPS

Technique:

1 Stand with the feet hip-width apart
2 Squat down (slight forward lean), with the arms straight and back
3 Jump off both feet in a forward direction (fig. 5.34)
4 Swing the arms through while doing this
5 Land on the balls of the feet and take-off again immediately
6 Repeat this for several jumps
7 Try not to jump too far or balance will be lost

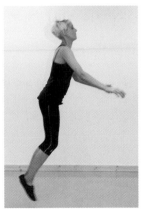

Fig. 5.34 Bunny hops take-off

BOUNDING

Technique:

1 Start off doing a slow jog
2 Slowly increase the pace
3 Make each step bigger and bigger until it feels like you are bouncing (fig. 5.35)
4 Swing the arms through while doing this
5 Land on the balls of the feet on each step and maintain balance
6 Try to maintain an upright posture
7 Aim for a short contact time of the foot with the floor

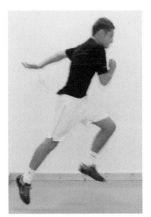

Fig. 5.35 Bounding

SINGLE-LEG HOPS

Technique:

1 Start with one leg in front of the other (fig. 5.36(a))
2 Jump forwards off the front leg in order to land on the same leg
3 Land on the ball of the foot and take off again immediately (fig. 5.36(b))
4 Swing the arms through while doing this
5 Bringing the opposite knee high will help
6 Repeat this for several jumps
7 Try not to jump too far or balance will be lost

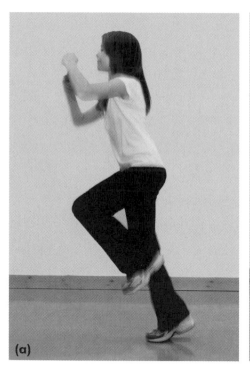 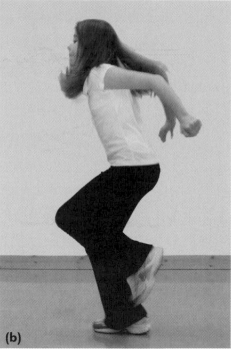

Fig. 5.36 Single-leg hops (a) Take-off (b) Transition

Upper-body plyometric exercises

MED BALL CHEST PASS

Technique:

- Start in the ready position with arms outstretched (fig. 5.37(a))
- The passer throws the med ball from a short distance (3–5 metres)
- On catching the ball, immediately cushion into the chest and throw it back (fig. 5.37(b))
- Try to speed up the transition

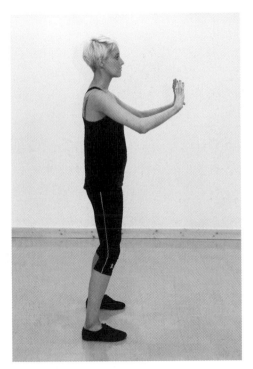 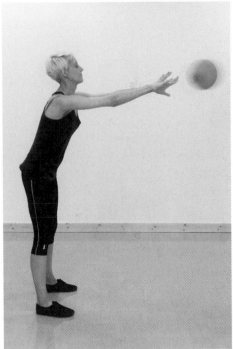

Fig. 5.37 Med ball chest pass (a) Ready position (b) Transition

MED BALL ROTATION

Technique:

- Start in the ready position with arms outstretched (fig. 5.38(a))
- The passer throws the med ball from a short distance (3–5 metres)
- On catching the ball, immediately bring the arms across the chest by rotating the upper body and throw it back (fig. 5.38(b))
- Try to speed up the transition

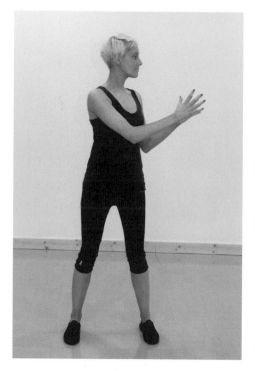 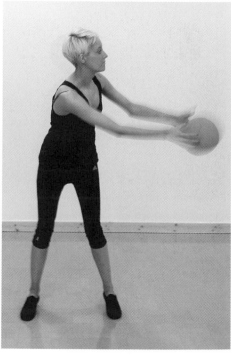

Fig. 5.38 Med ball rotation (a) Ready position (b) Transition

PRESS-UP BOUNCE

Technique:

- Start in the ready position with arms straight (figure 5.39(a))
- Lower the body quickly until the chest is about 5–8 centimetres off the ground then push up so that the hands leave the ground
- On landing in the press-up ready position, repeat the process again quite quickly (figure 5.39(b))
- Try to speed up the transition

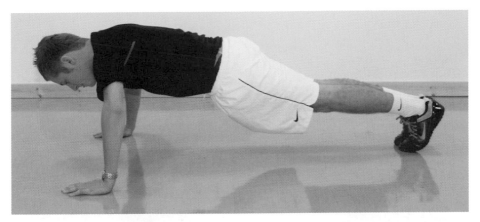

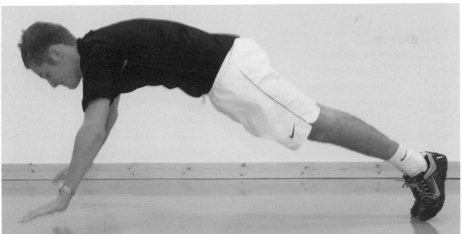

Fig. 5.39 Press-up bounce (a) Ready position (b) Transition

CHAPTER SIX
Qualities of a coach

Objectives

After completing this chapter the reader should be able to:

- Identify and discuss the qualities required for good coaching.
- List and describe various types of listening skills used in coaching.
- Discuss and give examples of different types of feedback methods that coaches can use.
- Explain the GET feedback method.
- List the types of communication skills under the headings 'verbal' and 'non-verbal' and discuss the benefits of each type.
- List the types of motivational skills under the headings 'intrinsic' and 'extrinsic' and discuss the benefits of each type.
- Discuss methods of good practice in relation to delivery of sessions.

Introduction

The list of qualities generally considered to be important for a coach to possess is endless; therefore, for the benefit of those new to coaching, we will focus on those qualities that are considered to be vital (there are many other important ones) to creating a good coaching environment for children. Figure 6.1 shows those particular qualities that have been chosen and explained in a bit more detail. However, the coach should understand that they need to read beyond this book to identify and improve other qualities which may be important in relation to their chosen sport or event.

Listening skills

It is commonly the case, not just in coaching, that most of us 'hear' but we don't 'listen'. For example, have you ever met anyone for the first time and within a few minutes you can't remember their name? Sounds familiar doesn't it? – I'm sure we have all done it. One of the reasons for this is that we often place more importance on what we have to say than on what others have to say. Generally speaking, there are two types of

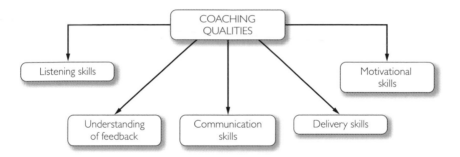

Fig. 6.1 Qualities of a coach

listening: passive and active.

- Passive listening: When we ask ourselves the question what 'listening' means, we often assume it is just the action of listening to what others have to say, without giving any kind of response. This kind of listening is otherwise known as 'passive listening'. Passive listening is generally considered to be fine in some situations, such as if you are watching a movie or listening to music, but in a coaching situation, how does the speaker (this could be the coach or the participant, i.e. the person taking part in the activity) actually know that the listener understands what is being said if they don't respond?

- Active listening: This type of listening is when a person listens to a speaker and responds in some way to show that they understand the speaker. In active listening, the coach might have to respond to questions or general statements from the participants, depending on the context or the situation. Just a few out of many possible coach's responses are given in the two example scenarios.

As you can see from both scenarios, responding to a participant's statement or ques-

Example 1: Question scenario

Participant question: 'Do you think I will play well today, coach?'

This seems like a fairly harmless question but participants often ask this because they need reinforcement and encouragement as their confidence is low and they are worried about failure. One way a coach could respond is by saying: 'As long as you try your best then I will be really happy.' In this way the coach is showing understanding of the question but reinforcing that losing is fine because it is the effort and participation that is important.

Example 2: Statement scenario

Participant statement: 'I think that I played really well today, coach.'

This statement requires a response by the coach to show understanding but the coach must consider the response carefully. For instance, the participant may not have played well so the coach may need to make the participant aware of this. In this scenario the coach could ask another question such as: 'Did you think all of your game was good, or were there things you think you could improve on?' This would show that the coach listened and would open up a debate to help the coach point out areas for improvement. If the participant did play well, in most cases they still need encouragement. In this scenario the coach could say: 'You did play well today but, tell me, is there anything you want to improve on for next time?' Again this shows understanding but challenges the participant to always try harder.

tion is not always as straightforward as it might seem. Coaches almost always have to interpret what has been said to them, as there is often an underlying message that the participant is trying to communicate. Experience of coaching and coming across these situations on a regular basis is invaluable in these cases, as each scenario can have many outcomes depending on the response of both the participant and the coach. The top tips for listening in table 6.1 might help the coach to improve their listening skills.

Table 6.1 Top tips for listening

1 As a coach you need to understand and accept that listening is important.

2 Listen and don't just hear. Focus on the speaker and concentrate.

3 Look for the underlying meaning or hidden message. As in the scenarios 1 and 2, is there a hidden message?

4 Try not to interrupt the speaker unless they are disadvantaging the rest of the group.

5 Think before responding. It is always best not to respond emotionally. Reflect for a few seconds if you need to.

Feedback skills

One of the simplest descriptions of feedback, in relation to the participants during activity or exercise, could be the way in which they acquire information from various sources to help improve the skills they are trying to learn. Some of the information (or relevant information to be more precise) can come from external sources, which is referred to as 'extrinsic feedback' and some can come from internal sources, which is referred to as 'intrinsic feedback'. Figure 6.2 gives some examples of both extrinsic and intrinsic feedback sources.

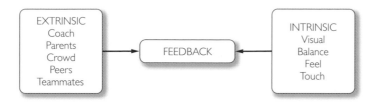

Fig. 6.2 Types and examples of feedback

- Extrinsic feedback: This simply means the participant gets information about the skill being practised from one of many different sources such as the coach or fellow participants. For example, a coach could make a comment to the participant about the standing foot placement when striking a football. Be aware, though, that there are often many confusing comments given to children by passive 'observers' during activity sessions or games. These observers quite often tend to be overenthusiastic parents, who sometimes get carried away and are not aware of what they are doing. In cases like this, be polite and ask observers to limit their comments to positive encouragement rather than tactical advice.

- Intrinsic feedback: This feedback, on the other hand, is related to the feelings and senses of the participant during a skill practice. Examples of this could be watching the flight of a ball when they try a slice shot, or how the grip felt during a forehand drive. It can be a good idea not to comment too much during practice and allow children to try to work out the skill using their own intrinsic feedback. This is sometimes called 'guided' or 'discovery' learning and is a method that coaches have found successful in many sports over the years.

Information overload

One of the reasons for not making too many comments in training or during games or events is that, as human beings, we are limited in the amount of information we can take in and concentrate on at any one time (this is due to the complex subject of short- and long-term memory processes, which will not be covered in this book). We are, however, capable of taking in more visual information (through sight) than verbal information. For this reason, it is important that the coach doesn't give too much verbal information

Table 6.2: Example of information overload

TRY THIS!
You will need enough pens and paper for the number of children in the group.

With a group of children you are coaching, give them all a pen and some paper. Read out a seven-digit number, get the children to wait for five seconds and then ask them to write down the number (they have to remember it obviously). Do this again but use an eight-digit number and ask them to write it down after a five-second wait. You should find that most of them will have written the seven-digit number down correctly but completely messed up the eight-digit number.

This is a phenomenon called 'chunking'. Very simply, if the brain thinks it will be overloaded it will tend only to remember the first and last bits of a piece of information.

during sessions and gives good quality demonstrations. Have a go at the exercise in table 6.2 to see for yourself the effect of verbal information overload on memory.

During the first stage of learning (*see* chapter 3), children need to think a lot about the skill, so coaches should be careful not to overload at this stage by giving too many coaching points or feedback. Coaches should try to work on just one or two skills at a time and allow children plenty of practice doing them.

Did you know
The word 'gaffer' is often used to refer to a coach. It comes from the shortened version of the word 'grandfather', used in the olden days as he was thought to be wise!

Giving feedback
Quite often children do not like to be singled out when coaches give feedback so a simple strategy that could be used is the GET 'general – eye contact – talk' feedback system, which is shown in figure 6.3. The GET feedback system has been devised as a simple method for relaying to participants information (not too complex) usually related to the performance of skills or techniques.

If a coach needs to make a feedback comment to one or two individuals about a skill during a group practice session, they should follow the GET feedback method. First they need to stop the practice and make the general (G) feedback comment to the whole group without looking at just the individual who the comment is directed at. By doing it that way, others in the group should not be aware of who the coach is talking about and, more importantly, it doesn't single out any individual. The coach should then restart the practice.

If the coach thinks that the general comment didn't work, they should stop the practice again. This time they should repeat the feedback comment and try to make eye contact (E) with the individual(s) in question at the same time, without being too obvious.

If that approach still doesn't work and the feedback appears not to have had any impact, the coach might have to talk (T) directly to the individual(s) concerned. If this last stage of the GET feedback system is used, the coach should try to do this quietly and without drawing attention to the individual(s). It would be sensible to do this without stopping the practice – most children

| GENERAL |
| Make the feedback comment to the whole group without looking at any individual |

↓

| EYE CONTACT |
| Repeat the comment but make eye contact with the individual |

↓

| TALK |
| Speak discreetly to the individual/s |

Fig. 6.3 The GET feedback system

will not be aware of what is going on as they would be too busy trying to concentrate on their own performance. The top tips for giving feedback in table 6.3 should help you to develop these skills.

Table 6.3 Top tips for giving feedback

1 Rather than using verbal instructions all the time, try to use visual demonstrations as often as possible because they will be remembered more easily.

2 Limit the amount of information at any one time if you must give verbal feedback. You will just lose the children otherwise.

3 Give feedback about the overall performance and not about the participant (i.e. avoid being judgemental).

4 Try to be consistent when giving feedback as children will always remember the previous time that feedback was given in a similar situation.

5 Use the GET feedback system (general – eye contact – talk) so as not to single out individuals.

Communication skills

In relation to coaching, the term 'communication' simply means a way of getting information across to the participants so that they can understand. In coaching there are two methods of communication that the coach can use: verbal (through the use of the voice) and non-verbal (by the use of gestures).

- Verbal: As we have discussed already, humans are not great at retaining much verbal information so it is wise to limit the amount that is given in coaching situations. It is also important for the coach to try to talk in a simple and clear way so that participants are not confused: the information provided should be at their level and not too complicated.

- Non-verbal: To communicate non-verbally just means getting your point across without speaking. Have you ever been on holiday to a country where you didn't speak the language but you managed to communicate by using all sorts of gesture? This just shows how effective non-verbal communication can be. This type of communication is sometimes called 'body language' and can be split into various categories as shown in table 6.4.

Table 6.4 Categories of non-verbal communication	
Category	**Description**
Role model	The way in which you look and dress can often influence children. If you do not look after yourself physically, it will give an indication to the participant that you are not bothered about fitness. Also, if you do not dress appropriately, this could have an effect on participants as well.
Body position	The way you position yourself with participants is very important. Don't get too close (in their personal space) as it could intimidate them. Also do not turn your back, as this is often construed as being given the 'cold shoulder'.
Body movements	Simple gestures with the eyes, hands, head etc. can be very effective. For example, a tilt of the head to the side with furrowed eyebrows can easily say 'Why did you do that?'
Voice	You will often have heard the saying 'It's not what you say but how you say it.' Children easily pick up on how we say things so avoid sarcasm.

Think of a coach who you admire and would like to emulate and you will probably think of someone who is a good role model for many reasons. Most likely they will always look the part and present themselves well but they will also be professional at all times. They are normally the first ones to congratulate the opposition and are gracious in defeat. If you respect them as a coach, it makes sense to try to gain respect from your own participants in the same way. Top tips for communication in table 6.5 might help you as a coach.

Table 6.5 Top tips for communication

1 Try to use a range of body language techniques to see if they work.

2 Pitch the information at the level of the participants when communicating verbally. Keep it simple!

3 Present yourself as a role model.

4 Ask other coaches to give you feedback on your own communication skills.

Did you know
Over 70 per cent of communication is non-verbal!

?

Motivational skills

As with the case of feedback, there are many different ways in which to motivate children in relation to exercise and activity participation and adherence, but the methods are generally grouped into two categories (*see* chapter 2): extrinsic motivation (from external sources) and intrinsic motivation (from internal sources).

Extrinsic motivation

Motivation of this category can come from many external sources such as trophies, badges, praise or other such rewards. These rewards can help to motivate younger children at the beginning but coaches should try to rely on this less and less as time goes on and foster conditions to build internal motivation. Children also value the comments of coaches and constantly look for praise at every opportunity. As with all young children, praise is a great motivational tool and can be used in many situations, such as in conjunction with giving corrective feedback. However, as a coach you will often have to correct actions or mistakes, and praise can help you to deliver this criticism. This method is called the 'criticism sandwich' and is a good way in which to deliver any corrections or criticism that you might want to make.

For example, you might need to give corrective information to a participant about their standing leg when they take a free-kick. The top slice of the sandwich would be to say something like: 'Good effort with that try'; the filling of the sandwich would be: 'Try to lean forwards when you strike the ball this time'; and the bottom slice of the sandwich: 'Just try your best'. In other words, the filling of the sandwich is the criticism and the slices of the sandwich just try to make it positive.

The other problem that faces the coach in relation to extrinsic motivation is what to praise and when to praise. Even though the range of situations in which this can occur is vast, table 6.6 gives some common examples of what a coach should praise and when he should do this.

Table 6.6 Typical examples of giving praise

What to praise	When to praise
Praise the performance and not the outcome – for example, if a participant hits a really good shot they have been working on but the opponent reacts well to it, the shot was still good!	Praise often and at the time with beginners – they need frequent praise, but do this just after they have performed a skill well so that they know it. This mainly applies to skills at the first stage of learning.
Praise effort and hard work – participants might work really hard but never win. Praising the hard work can often prevent the fear of losing or failure.	Praise occasionally for learned skills – once participants are at the autonomous stage of learning, praise should still be given but occasionally.
Praise good sportsmanship – this goes without saying. All sports need good role models who show sportsmanship.	Praise when deserved – the most important point is that you only give praise when it is deserved.

Intrinsic motivation

As opposed to external sources of motivation, intrinsic motivation is usually linked to the feelings or perceptions of the individual who is participating in the sport or event. Although this is a complicated topic, having fun, feeling competent and possessing a desire to win can all be classed as internal motivational factors.

Children who tend to be internally motivated are often driven by the need to succeed and to win, as they usually associate winning with success and losing with failure. For this reason, it is up to the coach to try to set targets and goals so that a reasonable amount of success can be achieved on a regular basis, especially with younger children. It can often be the case that if a child who is internally driven does not experience at least a small amount of success they are likely to blame themselves for the 'failure', thinking that they do not have the ability to be successful. There are, however, a small percentage of children who would use failure as the motivation to try harder because they thought that the failure was due to lack of effort. Not only does the coach need to create a successful environment for children like this but also they need to stress the importance of taking part and getting enjoyment out of participating.

In science, the internal drive to succeed is known as 'achievement motivation'. In other words, the theory surrounding achievement motivation suggests that the main motivation for individuals comes from the drive to succeed. In simple terms, this theory states that there are two main (and broad) categories of personality. The first is the category of those individuals who want to achieve success and the second is the category of those who want to avoid failure. Although this topic is much more complex, many coach educators agree that in the early stages of development it is best to try to develop and encourage intrinsic motivation. Figure 6.4 gives a quick visual reference of the differences between extrinsic and intrinsic motivation.

As a coach, try to be as positive as you can at all times since this kind of environment will help build self-esteem and confidence, whereas a negative attitude will only create a fear of failure and lack of self-esteem. That doesn't mean you are always praising and complimenting, as corrections can always be given in a positive manner as well. The top tips in table 6.7 should help you with regards to motivating your participants.

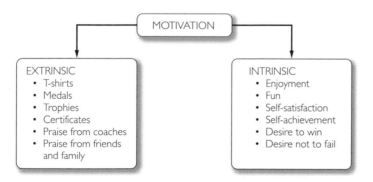

Fig. 6.4 Differences between extrinsic and intrinsic motivation

Table 6.7 Top tips for motivating

1 Use the criticism sandwich when trying to correct any action (praise – criticism – praise).

2 Give lots of praise to beginners in activities to help them develop.

3 Make sure that rewards are not given just to the winner. Reward hard work and fair play etc.

4 Try to be positive at all times to create an atmosphere to build self-esteem.

5 Only give praise when the participants deserve it.

6 Stress the importance of participation and taking part as well as winning.

7 Try to set achievable targets so that children can experience some level of success.

Delivery skills

As a coach, having knowledge and understanding of all the areas related to teaching exercise to children is irrelevant if your delivery skills are poor and not good enough to engage the children. There are many methods of delivery that can be used and most coaches will have their own preference.

The IDEA method

I prefer to use something I call the IDEA method of delivery as illustrated in figure 6.5.

INTRODUCE

This might sound straightforward, but introducing a skill to be learned can be difficult, especially in a team situation. If you are consistent in this approach, it will make it much easier in practice. For instance, use the same signal each time when you want

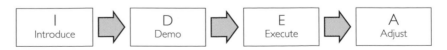

Fig. 6.5 The IDEA method of delivery

to get children's attention – this can be the use of a whistle or a command such as 'stop!'. Quite often they will be spread out so try to group them together rather than keep turning your head to address them all. If need be, have them sit down so that you can see all of them. Make sure, though, that the sun is at the back of the group of children so that they are not looking into it. Once they are in position you can introduce the new skill but keep this brief so that you can move straight to the demonstration.

DEMONSTRATE

As explained earlier in this chapter, try to limit the amount of talking and rely on visual demonstrations. It is crucial that you are able to demonstrate the skill correctly as the group will copy what you do – if you are not able to demonstrate, you should use someone who can. You may need to demonstrate more than once but don't take too long to do this, as you might lose the interest of the group. You should also demonstrate the skill at a slower speed than normal to give the group an adequate chance to observe it. Some coaches tend to give one or two main points before the group start practising the skill, but I prefer to just let them get on with it and make them aware of the points at a later stage.

EXECUTE

This is just another term for doing the practice. The group should be allowed to practise the skill as soon as possible after the demonstration. There are many different thoughts on how to practise, such as the whole-part-whole method where the skill is broken down into simpler parts and then put together again; however, the philosophy of multi-skills teaching, as in chapter 3, that skills should be taught progressively from simple to complex, doesn't really apply in this case. It is useful, though, to allow the group to experience some kind of success before moving on to another part of the activity.

ADJUST

This is just another term for correcting errors by giving feedback as covered earlier in this chapter. Practice alone is not enough for the group when developing skills, as they must receive some sort of feedback in order to progress to the next stage or skill. As with all verbal information, keep this to a minimum so as not to lose the attention of the group.

Assessing delivery skills

One way to try to improve on your delivery is to regularly assess your own performance. There are many ways in which to do this, such as peer assessment (getting your colleagues to assess your coaching). Table 6.8 gives an example of a self-assessment task for which you are asked to rate your own performance in different areas.

Table 6.8 Coach self-assessment

	1	2	3	4	5
My instructions are always brief and straight to the point.					
I always demonstrate correctly or use someone who can.					
I tend to give demonstrations from different angles so that the group can see.					
I never overcomplicate skills to be learned as I progress from simple skills.					
The feedback I give to participants is mostly positive.					
The feedback I give to participants is mostly visual.					
Most feedback I give is information about the skill and not judgement of the participant.					
I am usually quite consistent in the way I give feedback.					
I try to listen to what participants have to say as much as possible.					
I never single out individuals when trying to correct mistakes.					
I never reward just those who win. I always try to reward hard work as well.					
TOTAL					

In the self-assessment task, the more you agree with the statement the higher your score should be. Add up all the scores to give you a total. Generally speaking, the higher the overall score the 'better' the coach you should be. If you scored more than 33 points, you must have some good coaching habits. If you scored less than 33 points, maybe you should reflect on your coaching in order to try to improve. For instance, if you tend to give a lot of negative feedback because your participants need correction for their actions, are you setting your goals or expectations too high? Trying lowering your expectations – you never know!

CHAPTER SEVEN

Practical coaching

Objectives

After completing this chapter the reader should be able to:

- Discuss the priorities within a list of potential coaching objectives.
- List and briefly discuss a range of common coaching styles in relation to delivery.
- Explain the importance of planning for coaches.
- Discuss the importance of goal setting for coaches and describe this in the context of process and outcome goals.
- List and describe various methods used in coaching to identify components of fitness and skills.
- Discuss methods used by coaches to test components of fitness and specific skills.
- Define the term 'periodisation' and how this is broken down into phases or periods.
- Describe how different periods of the season can fit into a periodisation model.
- Discuss how methods can be used to periodise the various components of fitness.
- Explain the importance of regular testing.
- Identify and discuss the qualities required for good coaching.
- Discuss methods of good practice in relation to delivery of sessions.

Introduction

One of the main things anyone should consider, when thinking about coaching young children and young adults, is what they want to achieve or get out of coaching. Although there may be many reasons for the motivation to coach, the feedback from different coaches I have trained or with whom I have worked over the years (as well as from many coach education sources) tends to show that there are three main areas, or 'coaching objectives', that are commonly agreed upon. These main objectives are shown in table 7.1 and contain several priorities within each area.

Table 7.1 Main coaching objectives and priorities

Coaching objective	Priority
To help children win	• To put together a winning team • To help individuals win • To organise games and events so that teams or individuals can compete
To help children have fun	• To introduce children to fun activities • To de-emphasise competition and outcome • To allow children the chance to have fun and not to coach too much
To help children develop	• To develop fitness to participate in a variety of activities • To develop motor skills • To develop self-esteem, self-worth etc. • To develop socially

Obviously a coach cannot prioritise all the points within the main areas in table 7.1, as these priorities will often change depending on the situation of the coach and the group or individual they are coaching. However, it is often found that those coaches who prioritise winning tend to overemphasise the winning part and forget about the development of the participants. It is easy to sympathise with this particular viewpoint as society often rewards the winners and tends to neglect those who don't win (the so-called losers). Many coach educators are opposed to this viewpoint and agree that the participants being coached should always come first in any decisions that the coach makes and that the objective of winning should be secondary. If this approach does result in the team or the individual winning then it is a bonus; however, winning should still not be the main focus for young children. This is not to say that children should not try to win when they participate in activities. Trying to win should be encouraged but if a child isn't successful, they should be praised for their effort and commitment and encouraged to try to win another time. If children have the innate ability required to be successful in a particular sport or event, and the coach facilitates this by encouragement and positive coaching, then winning will more than likely be a consequence of their taking part.

Coaching styles

There are many ways in which people coach but perhaps the two most common coaching styles are those of 'autocratic' (do as I say) and 'democratic' (participants help in decision making). The autocratic coaching style can be further split into two types, 'telling' and 'selling', and the democratic style into 'sharing' and 'allowing'. Table 7.2 gives a visual overview of both styles and their respective types. Coaches do not normally use a single style of coaching throughout a session but often adopt a variety of styles or types depending on the coaching situation.

Table 7.2 Autocratic and democratic coaching styles and their types

Coaching style			
Autocratic		**Democratic**	
Telling	**Selling**	**Sharing**	**Allowing**
• Coach decides on what is to be done • Participants not involved in decisions • Coach defines what to do and how to do it • Participants told the exercises	• Coach decides what is to be done • Coach explains objectives • Participants encouraged to question and confirm understanding • Coach defines what to do and how to do it • Coach explains the object of circuit training and the purpose of each exercise • Participants ask questions	• Coach outlines training to the participants • Coach invites ideas from the participants • Coach makes decisions based on participants' suggestions • Coach defines what and how to do it • Coach identifies a circuit training session • Participants identify possible exercises for the circuit • Coach selects from the suggestions	• Coach outlines training to the participants • Coach defines training conditions • Participants explore possible ideas • Participants make the decision • Participants define what to do and how to do it • Coach identifies a circuit training session • Coach defines conditions of the circuit • Participants identify exercises for the circuit that meet the coach's conditions

These are not the only coaching styles by any means. For example, others have been suggested such as 'command' style and 'reciprocal' style:

- Command style is coaching where there is direct instruction and the coach makes all the decisions for the participants to follow. This style assumes that the coach knows what they are talking about so the participant listens.
- Reciprocal style (also known as 'cooperative style') is coaching where the participant takes some responsibility for their own development (although this is monitored and guided by the coach). Under the banner of reciprocal style, there are two different methods a coach can adopt: 'problem solving', in which the participant solves problems set by the coach, and 'guided discovery', in which the participant has freedom to explore various ideas or options.

Many people new to coaching adopt the command style. This can be because it is the style under which they themselves have been coached or because they can just dictate and avoid questions until they feel they are sufficiently knowledgeable. Unfortunately, the command style usually favours only the highly motivated athlete and doesn't really suit the majority of children who just want to participate and have fun.

The reciprocal style still allows the coach to guide and make decisions but it is up to the coach to make it look as though the participants have had a say in the decision-making process. It is not a problem for participants to make mistakes as long as they learn from them. This can be beneficial in many ways including having a positive effect on self-image. Regardless of what style of coaching is adopted, when working with children it is important (sometimes even more so than with adults) for the coach to have a plan of what they are doing and for any eventuality that may occur.

Planning a training programme

Coaches often question the need for a training plan or programme as it can be quite time-consuming to prepare and keep updated. There are many good reasons, however, why they should get into the habit of preparing one each time they undertake a period of coaching. If goals have been identified and agreed, the planning of training is vital so that the short-, medium- and long-term goals can be reached, providing the correct types of training activity have been put in place.

There are many different ways in which the coach can plan a training programme; however, many often follow the pathway identified in figure 7.1. The planning pathway is designed to work very simply. Before trying to devise any activities or training, the goals of the participant should always be discussed, irrespective of whether they are for performance or health or just for fun.

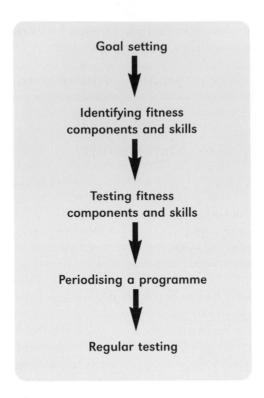

Fig. 7.1 Typical training planning pathway

Once the goals of the participant have been identified and agreed with the coach, the demands of the sport or activity should be identified. This is sometimes called a 'needs analysis'. For example, is there a lot of jumping involved by all participants? Does this involve jumping off one leg or off both? Once these demands are known, fitness components (*see* chapter 4) need to be identified that match the demands: for example, would good leg strength be needed for jumping? When the fitness components are identified, they must be put into some sort of order or programme, as it is important that some components are developed before others. For instance, leg strength would always be developed before trying to develop speed.

Finally, each component of fitness must be put into a comprehensive training plan (normally a minimum period of one year but depending on the goals) that shows when and which components will be developed and when testing of these components would take place. This overall planning is better known as 'periodisation'.

Goal setting

Although not used as often as it should be, goal setting is a simple technique that can provide important information to help structure a training plan. Goal setting can also provide a plan of action that can help the participant to focus on particular tasks. Regardless of the ability level, fitness status, experience or motivation of the participant, goal setting should be carried out and goals agreed by the coach and the participant as a negotiation process. Generally speaking, in relation to physical activity, goals can be split into two types, 'process goals' and 'outcome goals', as can be seen in table 7.3.

Table 7.3 Examples of process and outcome goals

Process goals	Outcome goals
• Be able to join in at tennis • Run or jog without pounding • Be able to do karate every week • Enjoy the activities that I do	• Reduce body fat • Win the county hurdles championship • Increase fitness • Complete a marathon • Reduce a dress size

Process goals are where the skill is broken down into manageable units that the participant can focus on. Often form or technique or simply participation can be classed as process goals as they are related more to just taking part than to results. Outcome goals are concerned only with the ultimate outcome, for example success or failure, or winning or losing. In other words, outcome goals are results-related as opposed to task-related. The coach should be wary that focusing too much on outcome goals can often affect attention to the process goals and result in a detrimental effect on the outcome, especially if the outcome goals are not achieved.

Goals can be set for the short, medium and long term depending on the participant and the type of activity. If only long-term goals were set, the participant might lose interest and adherence could be affected. Setting and achieving short-term goals could act as a motivational tool for the participant to help them progress to their next short-term goal. When agreeing goals with the individual, whether short-, medium- or long-term, the acronym SMART or SMARTER is a common guide for goal setting which includes several common characteristics that are often associated with effective goal setting. Table 7.4 gives an example of this.

Table 7.4 Examples of SMARTER goals (Honeybourne et al., 1998)

S	Goals must be *specific*	If an individual wants a weight-loss programme, be specific about the amount of weight that is set as the target. For instance, 0.5kg loss per week could be a specific target.
M	Training targets should be *measurable*	In the example above, 0.5kg is a measurable amount as opposed to 'lose a little weight' each week.
A	Goals should be *adjustable*	If an individual finds the target too easy or too hard, the coach must adapt the programme to suit. In other words, the programme must be adjustable.
R	Goals must be *realistic*	Set targets that are achievable. A 0.5kg weight loss per week is an achievable target for most people, whereas a target of over 3kg per week would not be achievable by everyone.
T	Training targets should be *time-based*	A 0.5kg weight loss per week can be a short-term target and can lead to an overall loss of about 26kg per year, which is a long-term goal.
E	Goals should be *exciting* (and challenging)	The chances of adhering to the programme are much greater if the programme is exciting in some way.
R	Goals should be *recorded*	Making sure that the individual keeps a record of exercise activity provides a visual stimulus for the individual and prevents any confusion over a longer term.

Identifying fitness components and skills

In order for coaches to provide a good training plan for a given sport, event or activity, the coach must know what the demands (in relation to fitness components) are. For the purpose of this chapter we will focus on the physical demands and skill components. Sometimes coaches will be working with individuals and sometimes they will be working in team environments. To understand the requirements of an individual participant within a team environment, a coach needs to know about the positional demands as well as the demands of the event. For example, in rugby, a back is regularly required to sprint distances of up to 50 or 60 metres, whereas a forward would typically sprint no more than 20 metres before being tackled. If the coach is not familiar with the positional, physical and skill demands of a particular activity, they would need to analyse the activity in some way to check this. There are many methods available to the coach for analysing activities and this is commonly known as a 'needs analysis'. Methods available include:

- Observational
- Video
- Player cam video
- Heart rate monitoring
- Fitness testing data

OBSERVATIONAL

For the majority of coaches, observational methods are probably the most commonly used form of analysis. Within this method there are many practices that range from making mental notes to recording observations using notepaper or computers. The type and amount of information collected during observations varies greatly between coaches as different methods suit different coaches. Whatever the method used, it is important that the coach considers the questions in table 7.5 beforehand.

Table 7.5 Observational considerations

Question	Consideration
Do you know what you are going to look for?	Are you counting the number of sprints, jumps, dives etc. or maybe the time spent sprinting, jogging or walking?
What is the best way to collect that information?	Are you using tick boxes for each item you are recording, or making general notes that there is a need for strength, power, speed etc.?
Do you know how you can use the information you have collected?	Are you going to base the training plan on this, or are you going to use the information again for comparison purposes or to check any progress?
Do you understand the limitations of the information you have?	Was the activity hampered in any way (e.g. weather conditions)? Did the athlete have a bad day etc.?

VIDEO
This is the relatively simple method of just videoing an activity and watching it back so that observations can be made at a later date. It is also useful to be able to stop the action while you are taking notes so that you don't miss anything. There are many problems associated with filming children (for obvious reasons), therefore the coach must familiarise themselves with procedures before doing so.

PLAYER CAM VIDEO
A player cam video is simply a video camera that tracks an individual player or participant for a certain period of time. Player cam tracks can be used to follow different participants at various intervals. For example:

- Player 1 tracked between 0–5 minutes and 15–20 minutes
- Player 2 tracked between 5–10 minutes and 20–25 minutes
- Player 3 tracked between 10–15 minutes and 25–30 minutes

An individual player can also be tracked throughout the entire period of the game or event rather than just for a short period of 5 or 10 minutes. A short period of tracking might not be representative of the contribution of the individual player during the whole game or event, as it may have been a poor period or a very good period. This method would obviously depend on the equipment that is available to the coach and on help to actually use the equipment during the game.

HEART RATE MONITORING
The heart rate of an individual can be checked by the use of a heart rate monitor (chest-strap and watch), which is better known as 'telemetry' or 'heart rate monitoring'. This method is used to assess the work rate or performance of an individual. One of the problems identified with heart rate monitors is that they sometimes experience interference from other electrical or magnetic sources such as overhead power-lines or measurements from adjacent monitors if they are close in proximity (normally just a few feet). In those individuals with a small chest, such as children or small-framed females, it may be difficult to achieve good contact and therefore heart rate measurements may periodically disappear.

In 2001, the company Polar introduced their Polar Team System to the sport and exercise market, which allows the collection of heart rate information from groups of participants. These systems are usually provided in sets of 10 monitors and cost in the region of £1000 to £2000, whereas a single monitor and watch would cost about £50.

FITNESS TESTING DATA
As a short cut for the coach, research has been conducted on the physiological demands of various sports and events and has provided useful data, as a result of fitness testing, that is even specific to a playing position within a particular sport. This type of testing can provide information known as 'normative data', which may be presented in tables

of average results usually collected for participants of different levels of ability normally grouped as elite, semi-professional or amateur, and separated by gender.

Testing fitness components and skills

Once the coach has carried out an analysis of the fitness components and skills required for a particular activity, they would then need to decide which components of fitness (see chapter 4 for more details) were important for the individual and which were only secondary. It is necessary to do this as the list of fitness components could be enormous and therefore unrealistic for the coach to then work with. Many experienced coaches would be able to do this without much help, but those new to this type of analysis could use a simple checklist template such as that in table 7.6, which has been completed for a midfield football player. It should be noted, however, that this type of analysis is largely subjective and different coaches might not agree on what is high, medium or low in terms of the importance of fitness components for a particular activity. By completing such a checklist, the coach would then be able to make an informed decision as to which fitness tests were suitable for the group that they were coaching.

Table 7.6 Components of fitness checklist

Component	Importance		
	High	Medium	Low
Cardio endurance	✓		
Muscular strength			✓
Muscular endurance		✓	
Flexibility		✓	
Balance	✓		
Speed		✓	
Agility	✓		
Power		✓	
Coordination	✓		
Comments:			

FITNESS TESTING

A range of fitness tests (or fitness assessments as they are commonly known) could be chosen on the basis of priority (such as testing those fitness components in the high-importance category first followed by those in the medium category if they were needed) but taking into consideration areas such as the availability of resources, the environment and the time availability. The implementation of any fitness tests for children is a huge and complicated topic and therefore beyond the scope of this book. However, table 7.7 gives an example of typical fitness tests that are commonly carried out in various sporting and event environments with young participants. The example, which is known as a 'physiological assessment sheet', has a column in which to record the results and another column that gives the target ranges relating to male and female groups based on data for specific age groups.

Table 7.7 Typical physiological assessment sheet

	Test	Test score	Target range	Comments
Body data				
	Height	cm	See BMI	
	Weight	kg	See BMI	
Body composition	BMI		Less than the 85th percentile	Based on age-related BMI charts for being overweight
Blood pressure	Manual blood pressure	mmHg	120/80 mmHg	N/A
Flexibility	Sit and reach test	cm	M: 20cm or above F: 30cm or above	Average or above for 16-year-olds

	Test	Test score	Target range	Comments
	Modified sit and reach test	cm	M: 14.5cm or above F: 14.5cm or above	Average or above for under 18 years of age
Endurance	Multi-stage fitness test	level	M: level 9.6 or above F: level 6.6 or above	Good or above for 13- to 19-year-olds
Balance	Stork test	s	M: 31s or above F: 16s or above	Average or above for 16- to 19-year-olds
Power	Vertical jump	cm	M: 50cm or above F: 41cm or above	Average or above for 15- to 16-year-olds
	Sprints: 15m 30m 40m	s s s	2.35s 4s 5.51s	N/A
Agility	Illinois agility test	s	M: 17.6s or less F: 22.4s or less	Average or above for 16-year-olds

Note: N/A = No comments on data available

In the list of selected tests in table 7.7 it should be noted that body data, body composition, blood pressure and flexibility are known as 'health tests' as they do not require any physical exertion of the subject being tested. The other tests are known as 'fitness tests'. The coach should be aware that there are many areas of knowledge relating to fitness testing that they should be aware of before trying to undertake any of the above tests. Areas such as reliability, validity and errors associated with testing are just some of the topics with which the coach should familiarise themselves. There is also the issue of making sure that conditions before, during and after testing have been addressed appropriately. These conditions are known as 'pre-test', 'during-test' and 'post-test' conditions. For more information relating to the underpinning knowledge of health and fitness testing, refer to *Practical Fitness Testing* (Coulson and Archer, 2009).

SKILL TESTING

Having tested the components of fitness that were chosen, the coach would then need to decide what individual skills were to be tested (for each individual as this could vary with position) and how to go about testing them. This list of skills would obviously be related to the particular sport or event. Because of the huge variation in possible sports (and indeed the skills within them), an example of those related to football has been done for you in table 7.8. These kinds of test are very subjective, which means that the coach rates the performance, in their opinion, of each skill (on a scale of 1–10 in the example given in table 7.8). These skill assessment sheets should be kept for comparison purposes at a later date. The assessment sheet is easy to use in that the coach observes particular individuals during a game situation and gives a score based on their own judgement.

Table 7.8 Skill assessment sheet

Skill	Score 1 2 3 4 5 6 7 8 9 10	Comments
Control		
Feet		
Chest		
Head		
Dribbling		
Right foot		
Left foot		
Running with the ball		
Passing short		
Right foot		
Left foot		
Passing long		
Right foot		
Left foot		

Skill	Score											Comments
	1	2	3	4	5	6	7	8	9	10		
Crossing												
Right foot												
Left foot												
Shooting and finishing												
Right foot												
Left foot												
Heading												
Defending & general												
Attacking												
Defending												
Tackling												
Preventing participants turning												
Closing down participants												

There may also be parts of the game, other than components of fitness and skills, that the coach wants to assess. One area that could be assessed relates to the individual's awareness of the game. This is often known as 'functional awareness' or 'tactical

Table 7.9 Functional awareness assessment sheet

Topic	Score											Comments
	1	2	3	4	5	6	7	8	9	10		
General												
Tactical awareness and appreciation												
Positional sense												
Awareness and vision												
Attitude and discipline												

Table 7.9 Functional awareness assessment sheet *(Continued)*

Topic	Score										Comments
	1	2	3	4	5	6	7	8	9	10	
Defending											
Defending as part of a unit: pressurising											
Defending as part of a unit: covering											
Tracking											
Patience and discipline											
Communication											
Accepting responsibility											
Possession											
Appreciation of maintaining team shape and pattern											
Creating space as an individual											
Creating space as part of a team plan											
Support play: readiness, timing and effectiveness of											
Forward runs: timing, quality and effectiveness of											
Accepting responsibility											

awareness' and, like all other areas, depends on the particular sport or event. An example assessment sheet that could be used for this purpose is shown in table 7.9 and could be used, for example, in football.

Periodising a programme

Long-term plans, or 'periodised training programmes' as they are known, were initially designed for use with athletes and were allegedly used by competitors in the months prior to the ancient Olympics. Perhaps the most recent recognised work relating to periodised programmes is that of Metveyev and Bompa in the 1960s.

The term periodisation is quite common among coaches and simply means planning or structuring a training programme. Within a programme, the coach caters for things such as the training variables (frequency, intensity, time and type) and components of fitness (cardiovascular endurance, muscular strength and endurance, flexibility and motor skills) for a specific time period. To further complicate the planning, the coach also needs to combine other areas such as technique, game or event strategy, nutrition and psychology.

Periodisation is often used for team games or athletes by dividing a season or yearly training plan into smaller, easier to manage, training phases or periods. Periodisation can often help an individual or athlete to achieve peak performance at the correct stage of the season, as it is often the case that doing the same training cycles continuously can lead to staleness and overtraining. Typical periods or training phases that are used by coaches are known as 'microcycles', 'mesocycles' and 'macrocycles'.

- A 'microcycle' is the name given to a short-term period of training sessions and for ease of use typically lasts for seven days (although this can vary). The short-term goals of each microcycle should be set in advance so that the coach and the participants know what they are doing. Microcycles can focus on many different factors such as endurance, speed, strength, technique and muscular endurance. The demand or load of each microcycle is determined by the number, volume and intensity of sessions within it. It is advisable to start each microcycle with a low- or moderate-intensity session and progress from there.
- A 'mesocycle' is a medium-term period and typically lasts between four and six weeks or longer: it should emphasise specific targets or components such as technique or speed. The length of the mesocycle is usually shorter as a competition or major event approaches, and the intensity of each microcycle within a mesocycle may vary considerably. Training components for mesocycles usually include basic conditioning, technique, speed, strength, hypertrophy and power.
- A 'macrocycle' is a long-term period that usually consists of two or three mesocycles. For sportspeople or athletes, a macrocycle is sometimes divided into three phases: the general and specific preparatory phase, the pre-competitive and competitive phase, and the transition phase. Team games refer to these phases as 'pre-season', 'in-season' and 'off-season'.

To help visualise how all the terms are related in an overall training programme, figure 7.2 gives an example plan for a typical team sport such as netball or football for a period of one year, although the coach must be aware that this is a flexible model depending on many factors such as cup competition success, weather and injuries.

Phase	Macrocycle				
	Pre-season		In-season		Off-season
	General	Specific	Peaking and tapering		Off-season
Mesocycle					
Microcycle					

Fig. 7.2 A typical one-year periodisation model

PREPARATORY PHASE

This particular phase of a training programme can last from as little as two months for team sports such as football and rugby to as much as six months for certain athletic events. There are also some sports, such as tennis, that don't have any specific preparatory phase as they last practically the whole year round. It is an important phase in a training programme, however, as it prepares the participants for the season to come. This phase is also sometimes split into two sub-phases: 'general' and 'specific'. The general sub-phase is normally used to develop general fitness as this normally follows a rest period for the participant. Once a certain level of general fitness has been achieved, the specific sub-phase would concentrate more on the specific demands of the sport or event.

PRE-COMPETITIVE AND COMPETITIVE PHASE

This is a difficult phase as the participants will be involved in matches or competitions. One of the most common problems associated with this phase is fatigue. This is mainly because of the difficulty in trying to fit training sessions into a schedule where the participant is playing matches or taking part in competitions. Recovery is crucial, especially for the young participant, and therefore the coach needs to be fully aware of this during periods when children are playing lots of matches or are taking part in many competitions. The 'juggling' act between recovery and training is known as 'peaking and tapering', which just means trying to reduce the training load (tapering) to recover enough (peak) for the competition ahead. Much research has been done on this and most agree that the best way to reduce the training load is to keep the same intensity of training at that time but reduce the amount of training (i.e. the training volume) by no more than about 40% and the frequency of training by no more than 20%.

Example
Reducing the training load during tapering

If a coach had prescribed cardiovascular training of 10km runs at a frequency of five times per week, then during tapering this could be reduced to 6km runs at a frequency of four times per week (but no fewer than this).

TRANSITION PHASE
This is the phase when the participant does not take part in any training or competitions and essentially has a break to fully recover ready for the preparatory phase. Adults would normally be advised to do light training in this period just to maintain a certain level of fitness but this advice is not necessary for children, who tend to be active anyway.

There are many components of fitness (*see* chapter 4) that the coach might want to develop; therefore, they would need to be addressed in the periodised programme. This is a very complicated process but for the purpose of this book, as a starting point for the beginner new to coaching, it will be split into two areas: cardiovascular periodisation and strength and endurance periodisation.

CARDIOVASCULAR PERIODISATION
Periodisation for athletes doing events is often different from periodisation for participants doing team sports. In the case of athletes doing events, one of the more common ways of periodisation used is the 'training pyramid' method. If we think about cardiovascular training as that in which the heart rate increases from a lower level to a higher level over a period of time, the cardio training pyramid in figure 7.3 will help to visualise this.

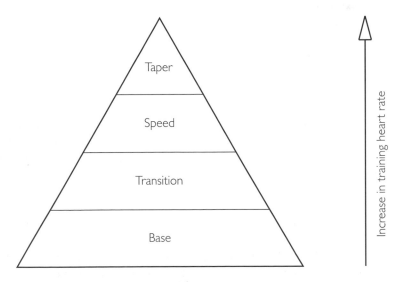

Fig. 7.3 The cardio training pyramid

This type of training model involves doing several months of 'base-work'. This simply means relatively high-volume but low-intensity cardiovascular training in order to develop good aerobic endurance. The difficulty for the coach is knowing how long to continue this type of training. One way to help determine this is to monitor the performance of the participants on a regular basis. If no increases in performance are seen to occur, it is usually an indication that it is time to move on to the next stage of training. This stage is known as 'transition training': it usually lasts for about four weeks and involves lower volumes of training (fewer km), but at higher intensities (around the anaerobic threshold as explained in chapter 4). The next stage of cardio training is usually to focus on speed. It is typically done at high intensities and low volume but only lasts for a period of between two and three weeks.

Finally, there is the 'taper' stage, which is very important: this is used as preparation for competition and normally lasts between 24 hours and three weeks depending on the sport. Essentially this means cutting down on the amount of training to try to totally recover from any fatigue the participants might be suffering from. It is often difficult to get participants to taper due to their fear of losing fitness, but a correctly applied tapering strategy has been shown to improve performance by up to 3% (for more information on tapering see earlier in this chapter).

For participants in team sports, a simple graph of volume and intensity is often used for periodisation. Figure 7.4 gives a very general overview of how volume and intensity of cardiovascular endurance training could vary over a one-year macrocycle and how skills training could fit into this.

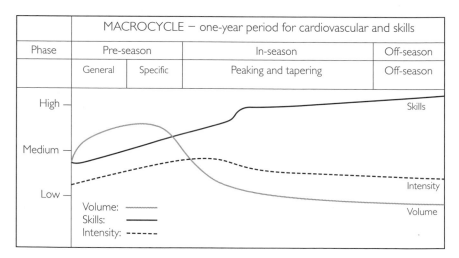

Fig. 7.4 General periodisation of cardiovascular endurance in terms of volume, intensity and skills

It should be noted that the skills component training in figure 7.4 would be a lot less for adults than for children due to factors such as boredom. As can be seen in figure 7.4 the amount of cardiovascular training in pre-season would build up to be quite high, with the intensity starting off low and then building up as well. The idea would be to build up to peak cardiovascular fitness ready for the start of the season and, as the season starts, to try to maintain this. The volume of training tends to reduce considerably during the in-season due to matches being played. During the off-season, the volume of training is reduced to a 'tick-over' level, keeping the intensity at a minimum.

STRENGTH AND ENDURANCE PERIODISATION

Muscular strength and endurance is a component of fitness that tends to be periodised for adults but is not often addressed for children. In effect, for adolescents, the type of periodisation would be the same but the intensities would be much less than those for adults. One theory or model that is used to plan resistance training is called the 'step-loading' model. This model is much easier to visualise in a building-block style as shown in figure 7.5.

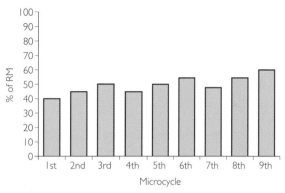

Fig. 7.5 Example of a step-loading model for resistance training

Simple progressive overload training programmes are often thought to be boring and repetitive for the individual, as well as leading to staleness and increasing the risk of repetitive loading injuries. The opposite is true with step-loading programmes, which are thought to decrease the risk of repetitive injuries and be less boring. Step-loading models normally include two or three short cycles (microcycles) of increased intensity followed by a short cycle of decreased intensity (similar in intensity to the second cycle) before repeating the process again. In the example in figure 7.5, the intensity is prescribed by percentage of RM and it can be seen here that short cycles of specific intensities can be performed in sequence. The cycles could represent microcycles of a week in duration. The coach should note, however, that the intensities are just examples and in practice will depend on many variables relating to the individual and the event for which they are training.

The step-loading model could also be thought of in terms of low-, moderate- and high-intensity cycles that increase in intensity when repeated. Quite often these cycles are a week long and accumulate over a set part of the season. The moderate-intensity training week is usually representative of an average training week and the low- and high-intensity weeks are adjusted to this level. This is just one way that resistance training can be programmed and the example in figure 7.5 assumes that participants have little resistance training experience and therefore the loads are kept quite low.

A step-loading model can be used for the majority of team participants of a young age. However, for coaching older children who are competing in athletic events a slightly different model can be used, in this case known as the 'resistance training pyramid' model shown in figure 7.6.

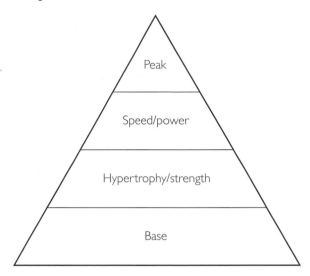

Fig. 7.6 The resistance training pyramid for children over the age of 12 years

As with all resistance training programmes and especially with children, a period of training known as 'base conditioning' should be done to prepare the athlete for more strenuous training. At this base stage the athlete should train using only moderate loads (12–15RM for example). This stage should last for only a few weeks for those athletes that have some sort of resistance training experience. However, the stage should last up to a few months for those that have had little or no experience of resistance training. One of the reasons for this is that the brain has to 'learn' the resistance exercises because they are relatively new as well as the muscles having to adapt to them.

The next stage in the pyramid would depend on the requirement of the sport or event: whether the athlete needed to 'bulk up' or not. If they did need to bulk up, moderate to high loads (6–12RM for example) with a moderate volume (3–5 sets for three sessions per week) of training would be done in order to develop muscle mass (for those who have an event requirement). For those athletes that just needed to develop strength, training with high loads (8RM or less for example) with a low volume for an initial period of about three to six weeks would be recommended, followed by a more challenging period of strength training.

Once a good level of strength was achieved by the athlete, power or speed training would then normally be done, again depending on the requirement of the sport or event. For power training, moderate loads are normally used but the repetitions tend to be done as quickly as possible. In this type of training the coach should also make sure that complete recovery is allowed between the sets. To develop speed, repetitions of light to moderate loads are performed quickly but this time with incomplete recovery between sets.

The demands of the event should always be analysed so that resistance training can match the demands. For instance, road cyclists need to have muscular endurance to cope with the hours of cycling but they also need power so that they can sprint in the final stages. The coach would therefore need to develop not only muscular endurance by training with many repetitions at light loads but also power using slightly heavier loads.

Peak training is just another term for a period when the training is made very specific to the demands of the sport or event.

Regular testing

The importance of regular testing should never be underestimated, as it provides the coach (and the person being tested) with valuable and varied information. There are many other important reasons why fitness testing is considered to be beneficial for both children and young adults (*see* table 7.10). One of the main reasons is that, as in the case of adults, testing can help to identify the ongoing effects of a training programme specific to an individual. This is useful as the testing results can help to make adjustments to the programme if necessary.

Some of the tests that are available may indicate potential problems, such as lower than normal flexibility or a lung function below the normal range, that should be investigated further by appropriately qualified personnel. This would act almost as a screening tool (*see* chapter 9) to help identify any possible impairments or conditions of the individual as early as possible. Other important benefits include motivation: an example of this would be the coach setting targets for the individual in certain tests (targets are normally based on previous tests). This is often a good motivational tool as individuals can then try to achieve the set targets (as long as they are achievable and have been agreed).

Table 7.10 Benefits of fitness testing

Benefit of testing	Description
Programming	Testing can help to establish an overall picture of physical condition. It also provides a starting point on which to base training programmes.
Screening	Testing can help to identify any particular problems that the coach needs to make aware to qualified people such as GPs.
Progress monitoring	By repeating tests at regular intervals, the coach will be able to see if individuals being tested are progressing or not.
Grouping	Testing can provide information which allows the coach to put participants into groups according to their ability.
Education	Testing can help to provide a better understanding, for both the coach and the participants, of the demands of the particular sport or event.
Assessing recovery	Testing is a very useful way to assess the recovery from any injuries that participants might have had and tell the coach if the participant is ready to start training again.
Motivation	Test results are often a good method to use to set standards and to motivate participants as they always like to try to beat their previous score.
Goal setting	Testing can be useful for setting short- and long-term goals and training programmes can be adapted using the test information.

CHAPTER EIGHT
Multi-skills activities

Objectives

After completing this chapter the reader should be able to:

- List and describe the components of a typical multi-skills session.
- Discuss relevant information related to the duration and intensity of warm-up, dynamic stretching, multi-skills main activity, cool-down and static stretching components.
- Describe the key points for delivery of each of these components.
- List various factors required for session planning.
- List typical areas for general delivery.

Introduction

The focus of this chapter is on giving practical guidelines for the delivery of multi-skill activity sessions as these movements provide the foundation of all sports and events. As with all activity sessions, multi-skills activities can be delivered either through after-school clubs in possible collaboration with extended schools or within school curriculum time (50% of primary schools must have had an extended school day by 2008 and 100% of primary schools by 2010). The activities are designed to be delivered at least twice per week for one hour from a skill-acquisition perspective.

The multi-skill activities in this chapter focus on participation rather than on end product, and have been designed for this purpose. The activities are progressive in nature and have been numbered in sequence for the coach to follow. It is important that skills are revisited from time to time and therefore a guide on how to programme for this will be given later in this chapter.

Multi-skills activity sessions

Every activity session a coach delivers will be different due to many factors that could influence the session such as the conditions, the environment or injuries. A good coach is always flexible in that they should be able to adapt the session; however, sessions should follow a similar pattern in relation to the components of the session. A typical multi-skills activity session is structured as in figure 8.1 in order of its components.

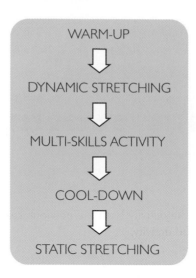

Fig. 8.1 Typical multi-skills activity session components

Warm-up

The component known as the warm-up is something that is always done at the start of an activity session and it is exactly what it sounds like. For all activities, it is essential that the body is fully warmed up. One of the main reasons for this is to reduce the potential for injury before starting the main activity (multi-skills in this case). This is because a great deal of research has shown that perhaps the main factor in muscular injury prevention is muscle temperature, as muscle is more elastic when warm and therefore will stretch more easily without damage. In other words – you risk fewer injuries when the muscles are warm! (To be precise, it is the tendon tissue that doesn't stretch well before it is warmed up and it is this tissue that is usually damaged.)

In relation to the warm-up it is important to understand how long and how hard it should be: its duration and intensity.

- Duration: The time period recommended for the warm-up is dependent on the environment and other factors but is usually at least five minutes. For instance, if the weather is hot, the warm-up time should be reduced as coaches should always bear in mind that children generally warm up much quicker than adults (*see* chapter 4). If the weather is cold, however, it makes sense to extend the warm-up period, even if this encroaches on the time allowed for the main activity.
- Intensity: The warm-up should be designed to stimulate the entire muscular system into a state of readiness, as well as warming the muscles; therefore it is suggested that an activity from the previous multi-skills session be used as the warm-up for the session to follow. It should be done at a walking or gentle pace, increasing the intensity until the children feel warm. This also acts as a refresher for the movements

taught previously, thereby enhancing the learning ability. As a general rule, the intensity of the warm-up should gradually increase to the level at which the main activities are intended to start.

When it comes to warm-up exercises, coaches can be inventive, which is always a good thing; however, try to use the warm-up key points below for each session so that the children become accustomed to the practice. There are several examples of typical warm-up activities at the end of this chapter.

WARM-UP KEY POINTS

- Start each session with the activity from the previous session.
- Demonstrate the warm-up activity.
- Get the children to do the activity at a walk or gentle pace.
- Gradually increase the pace of the activity.
- Get the children to do any movement activity at a jogging pace for one minute continuously, then ask the children how they feel (body temperature, heart rate and breathing).
- Move on to the next stage of the session when you think *all* children are warm.

Example warm-up sessions

1. Copy cat

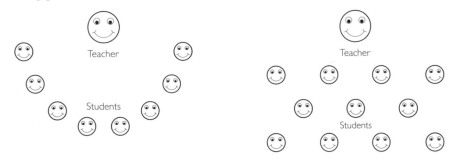

Direction
The idea is to demonstrate various on-the-spot and travelling movements so that children can copy you. Start with on-the-spot movements such as marching, twisting, bending etc. and progress to multi-directional movements such as marching, jogging, skipping etc.

Remember
- Make sure the children can see you at all times.
- Gradually build up the intensity of the movements.
- Make sure that there is enough space between children to allow for moving about.
- Return to the same spot after moving around.

2. Trains

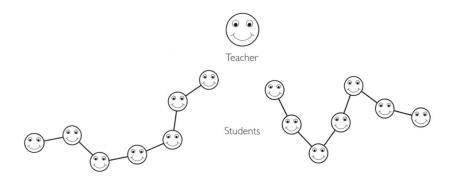

Direction
Split the class into smaller groups. The idea is to get each group to link hands and move around the room without crashing into each other. Start with slow movements and build up to jogging pace. Introduce items such as coming into a station where the children have to stop and do movements such as squatting or lunging, ready to go off again. The train could also slow down (going up hill) and speed up (going down hill).

Remember
- Make sure the children can see you at all times.
- Gradually build up the intensity of the movements.
- Frequently swap the linking hands.
- Do not allow the trains to go across each other.

3. Jungle trail or animal magic

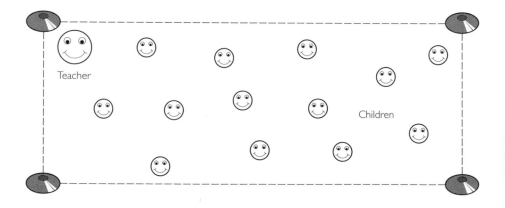

Direction

Put cones around a suitably large enough area. The idea is to get the children to act out the story of an adventure through the jungle. Ask them to imagine they are fighting through the undergrowth, trying to walk through thick mud, climbing trees, using stepping stones across rivers, swinging on vines, and so on.

Alternative

Get children to imagine they are animals such as chickens, tigers, elephants and so on and mimic the movements that are typical of these animals.

Remember

- Make sure the children can see you at all times.
- Gradually build up the intensity of the movements.
- Allow children to come up with scenarios.
- Make sure children have space around them.

Dynamic stretch

The common belief of many coaches is that stretching can reduce the risk of injury but it is often confusing as to which type of stretch, or indeed if any at all, should be performed, prior to any exercise or activity. It is therefore important to understand the difference between static and dynamic stretching exercises (*see* chapter 5 for a more in-depth explanation of this subject). In simple terms, dynamic stretching relates to stretching in motion where the contraction of a particular muscle is used to stretch the opposite muscle. This type of stretching is associated with how easily the movement can be done and not with the range of motion. The research relating to dynamic stretching is still in its infancy even though there are many books on this subject.

It is recommended to perform this type of stretch before the main activity as the stretches can closely mimic the activities to follow. Dynamic stretching can therefore form part of the warm-up if the coach wishes. Certain dynamic stretching exercises can be done in relation to sports-specific movements (by mimicking the movement but at a slower, more gentle pace) or general whole-body movements can be performed, such as those suggested in figures 5.11 to 5.18 in chapter 5.

- Duration: It should only take two or three minutes to do dynamic stretches if they are to be done after the warm-up; if they are included, the entire warm-up should last about 5–10 minutes.
- Intensity: Dynamic stretches should always be performed under control and not too quickly. The intensity should build up slowly so coaches should put stretches of this type in order of increasing intensity and gradually raise the pace at which they are performed.

As with the other components of the session, the coach should follow the key points below with regard to delivery of dynamic stretches but still be inventive with their chosen exercises.

DYNAMIC STRETCH KEY POINTS

- Incorporate these stretches into the warm-up or perform them just after as a separate session.
- Arrange the exercises in order of intensity.
- Start with small movements and gradually increase the range.
- Start with slow movements and gradually increase the pace.
- It helps to perform the stretches in an order such as from head to toe or from toe to head.
- The stretches can be performed to music, which can often help children to adapt quickly to the movements.
- Encourage precise execution of the movements.
- Choose the stretches relevant to the sport or activity that children will do in the main session.

Multi-skills activity

This is the main part of the session that follows on from the dynamic stretch component (or the combined warm-up/dynamic stretch component if they are done together). In this activity the main focus is on the skills that are being taught and the children having fun; however, the coach can still take into account any components of fitness (*see* chapter 4 for more details) on which they have planned to work, even though this might be a secondary focus of the session. In other words, sessions are based on a multi-skills theme but you should remember that variety and *fun* are the key.

There are example activity cards provided at the end of this chapter that explain how to deliver each session – these are just examples of some of the many multi-skills activity sessions that can be delivered. Coaches themselves should identify all the possible skills that can be taught (*see* chapter 7) and use their imagination to incorporate these skills into their own activity sessions. At the start of the multi-skills component, it is necessary to demonstrate the activities to the children: frequent demonstrations have been shown to increase learning but you need to make sure that they are executed correctly (*see* chapter 6 for more details).

- Duration: Main activity sessions should never be too long for younger children in order to prevent boredom and reduce the risk of fatigue. If sessions are kept short, it is likely that children will want to come back again. A duration of between 20 and 40 minutes is recommended for this type of activity.
- Intensity: This is entirely dependent on the aims of the session and the fitness/skill level and age of the participants and therefore coaches will need to read the other chapters in this book to familiarise themselves with the rationale behind setting the intensity levels.

MULTI-SKILLS ACTIVITY KEY POINTS

- Always start with a demonstration at a slow or gentle pace.
- Gradually increase the pace of the activity but encourage accuracy.
- Try to include vigorous (high-intensity) exercise at some point.
- Teach the children that they can go faster over shorter distances.
- Ask the children if they can tell the difference in the body between gentle and vigorous exercise.
- Ask the children to listen to others breathing.
- Ask children to identify the movements of others taking part. Use both dominant and non-dominant arms and legs, otherwise participants will lead with their preferred side.
- Limit the time that children spend in high-intensity activities. Break up the task by giving feedback at regular intervals.
- Try not to have sessions longer than 40 minutes in total.

Cool-down

As with the warm-up, the cool-down is a component that is also exactly what it sounds like. For instance, the main activity component will include periods of a vigorous nature that increase the heart rate levels of the children. For this reason, it is important that a cool-down period of low-intensity activity is given in order to return their heart rate to near-resting levels (or until the children appear to have recovered).

Although there are many other benefits of doing a cool-down component, research has shown that it can help reduce the 'stiffness' feeling that occurs in the days following intense exercise activity. Another advantage of doing a cool-down is that it can help the blood return to the heart after exercise. The reason for this is that if exercise stops suddenly, the heart is still beating fast and pumping lots of blood, which builds up in the lower legs (this is known as 'blood pooling') and has difficulty getting back to the heart (a process known as 'venous return'). Moving around and gradually reducing the heart rate has been shown to prevent this from happening.

- Duration: The cool-down can be of varying duration depending on the environment and intensity level of the main activity. For instance, if the main activity component was high-intensity, the cool-down would take longer. If the main activity was just low-intensity, the cool-down would be shorter. As a guide, the cool-down will be between three and ten minutes depending on the intensity of the main activity, but coaches must also take into consideration the temperature of the environment.
- Intensity: The whole point of doing the cool-down is to try to gradually reduce the heart rate levels so that the heart is not pumping lots of blood around the body. The cool-down intensity should start from the point at the end of the main activity component and gradually reduce in intensity until children have recovered to near-resting levels.

COOL-DOWN KEY POINTS

- Gradually decrease the intensity of the activity.
- Use the exercises that were used during the main activity but at a slower pace.
- Ask the children how they feel (body temperature, heart rate, breathing).
- Ask the children to listen to others breathing.
- Keep moving to avoid blood pooling.
- Finish the cool-down only when you think *all* children have reduced their heart rate levels and recovered.
- Perform static stretches at the end after recovery.

Cool-down activities can simply be made up of the skills that were practised during the main activity component but at a gradually reducing intensity. This could also help to reinforce the skills that were being taught.

Static stretch

Following on from the discussions in earlier chapters and various guidelines, it is recommended that static stretches be performed after the cool-down component. It makes sense that the heart rate has recovered so that there isn't a large amount of blood being pumped into a muscle when it is being stretched. It also makes sense that the muscles are being stretched after the entire activity session when they are at their warmest, which makes them more pliable (stretchy).

Although the benefits of static stretching for children are a hotly debated topic, getting them into a regular stretch routine or habit is a good idea as it will probably continue through to adulthood, when the need for maintaining flexibility is important. If the weather is not good and conditions are cold or wet, it is advised to do the static stretching component indoors to gain any benefit. Otherwise, children may end up negatively associating stretching with bad weather conditions.

- Duration: Static stretches are recommended following the cool-down in order to try to return the muscles to their original pre-exercise length. Guidelines state that stretches should normally be held for between 10 and 30 seconds and each one performed two or three times: for children, however, holding stretches for about 15 seconds would be fine. If stretches are compounded (done together), it should take no more than three or four minutes to complete this component.
- Intensity: It is difficult to give an intensity level for stretching as it depends on the children and their perceptions of how the stretch feels. Guidelines state that stretches should be held at the point of mild discomfort, which probably means nothing to children. Coaches should use phrases such as 'just until you start to feel the muscle stretch' or 'just where it gets a little tighter', but they should make sure that children understand that at no time should any pain be felt during a stretch.

STATIC STRETCH KEY POINTS

- Only stretch when children are fully recovered.
- Start with standing stretches and finish with seated or lying ones.
- Go straight from one stretch to the next and do not take longer than four minutes for this component.
- Only stretch outside if the weather is good.
- Hold each stretch for about 15 seconds and perform it two or three times.
- Make sure children understand that they should not feel any pain during the stretches.
- Focus on the stretch technique, which should improve as children get older.
- Make stretching a regular routine.

Planning multi-skills sessions

In chapter 7 we looked at periodising programmes: that gave an overview of how to structure programmes over a fairly long period of time. For many different reasons, the coach should also have a plan of each individual session that they do. Just putting together the session plan might jog the memory of the coach about something that they may have forgotten to do. The plan can also be used during the session itself in case the coach has a memory lapse and forgets what is coming next (we have all been in that situation). Session plans are individual and most coaches have their own version but table 8.1 gives an overview of the areas that should be included as a minimum.

Table 8.1 Items to include in an activity session plan	
Plan item	**Explanation**
Date	You may need to refer back to the plan to see on what dates you did certain activities.
Venue details	This would include address, telephone number, venue contact name, indoor/outdoor facility, disabled access, toilets, changing facilities, parking and spectator facilities.
Resources	You will need a full list of the equipment you need for the session such as balls, nets, cones, bibs and water bottles.
First-aider	Make sure you record the name and contact number of the venue first-aider at the time that the session will be delivered.

Table 8.1 Items to include in an activity session plan *(Continued)*

Plan item	Explanation
Session aims	The overall aim or aims of the session should be stated bullet-point style, for example: ● arm drive when running and one-handed catching.
Activity plan	You should have an ordered plan of your session from the introduction and warm-up right through to the cool-down, preferably with time allocations for each component.
Plan B	Always have a backup plan (even if it is just a brief note) in case of scenarios such as bad weather or running out of time.
Evaluation box	As a coach it is a good habit to evaluate each session that you deliver (as soon as you can after the session is finished) to give you an idea of how the session went for development purposes.
Action plan	If anything in the session could be improved, an action plan box is ideal for making notes that you can refer back to.

Some coaches may prefer to do their own session plan or have their own format that they use each session. Figure 8.2 gives an example of a simple session plan that you can use as is or adapt to suit your coaching style or situation that you are involved in. Some of the session plan has been filled in to give you an idea of how the template could be used.

Date:

Venue: Contact no: First-aider:
Contact no:

Session aims

This is a 45-minute session designed to teach the mechanics of running and hopping to a group of twelve under-14 male basketball players in a pre-season period. The team plays in a county league and all players have been with the team for at least two years. The main teaching points for the skills will be body position, arm swing, foot placement on landing and control of balance.

Plan B

Indoor hall is available in case of bad weather. The indoor facility could also be used for short conditioned games if needed. If the drills are too complicated, foot ladders are available for the same drills. If drills are too easy for the players, angled agility hop drills and target hop drills could be used.

First-aid point: Water:

Fire exits:

Equipment required:

Fig. 8.2 Example of a multi-skill session plan (continued on pages 194–196)

Time (min)	Component set-up	Teaching/coaching points
0–5	*Warm-up* Cone off a square 20m x 20m. Players to stand on one side of the square in a line.	Choose one of the warm-up activities from the list or have players inside the square doing ball drills at a gradually increasing pace.
5–8	*Dynamic stretch* Use coned-off square as above. Players start in line on one side of the square.	Use selected dynamic stretches from the list (chapter 5). Demo each stretch then have players perform each stretch in a line across the 20 metres of the square and then back again. Repeat this process but increase the pace of each stretch. Focus on the technique and reinforce teaching points of each stretch.
8–18	*Main activity* Place 2 rows of 8 hurdles in a straight line 0.5m apart. Split players into 2 groups or teams.	Demo peg-leg run. Each group perform one run at slow pace keeping good distance between players. Reinforce running leg skimming the hurdle and repeat run. Increase the pace but check technique. Do 4 or 5 runs then swap running leg and repeat the process.
18–22		In teams, have a peg-leg relay race. All players stay seated until they are high-5'd by the runner in front. Twice through (one on each leg) but only for fun (no teaching points).
22–32	Place 2 rows of 8 hurdles in a straight line 0.5m apart. Split players into 2 groups or teams.	Demo hopping over hurdles on take-off leg. Each group performs one run at slow pace keeping good distance between players. Reinforce landing on the ball of the foot and swinging the arms through. Increase the pace but check technique. Do 4 or 5 runs then swap hopping leg and repeat the process.

Fig. 8.2 (continued)

Time (min)	Component set-up	Teaching/coaching points
32–36		In teams, have a hopping relay race. All players stay seated until they are high-5'd by the runner in front. Twice through (one on each leg) but only for fun (no teaching points).
36–41	*Cool-down* Use the coned-off square with players lined up on one side.	Repeat the peg-leg runs but keep the players moving at all times. Gradually reduce the intensity and the pace and finish at a walking pace.
41–45	*Static stretch* Use coned-off square or indoor facility if weather is not good.	Select static stretches from the available list in order of standing to seated and upper body to lower body. Hold stretches for 15 seconds and do each one twice, reinforcing technique at all times.

Session evaluation

My strong points: The management of health and safety was very good. A risk assessment was carried out prior to the lesson to minimise the danger of causing injury. Rules were also agreed at the start to make sure that there was no gum being chewed or jewellery being worn at any time throughout the lesson. I felt the overall organisation of the skills was good in terms of setting up different drills in relation to the game situation and keeping to the timing of the session.

My weak points: With regard to instruction, I did not emphasise the correct technique on a regular basis and allowed the drills to continue too long between feedback comments. Although my demonstrations were technically precise, I mentioned nothing about which foot to put forwards first (should have been the dominant foot).

Fig. 8.2 (continued)

Fig. 8.2 (continued)

> **Action plan**
>
> I could try to make the lesson more challenging since some pupils progressed very quickly, leaving them unchallenged at times. Future lessons can be improved by giving feedback comments on a more regular basis and by informing players that it is OK to ask questions at any time if they don't understand, before they go away to try to do what was asked of them.

Although my top tips appear throughout this book, there are general delivery tips relevant to multi-skills activities that the coach should try to address at all times. Table 8.2 lists the general tips that are reinforced on many occasions in other chapters.

Table 8.2 General delivery tips	
1	Group the participants according to size and ability – *not* just age.
2	Take regular water breaks as children heat up quickly and sweat a lot.
3	As cardiovascular endurance is lower than in adults, restrict the duration of the activity to shorter than you would for adults.
4	Avoid excessive high-impact and repetitive actions.
5	Be aware of 'mood' and other psychological issues due to hormone levels.
6	Cater for gender differences.
7	Use the GET correction procedure – general comment, eye contact, talk direct.
8	Get children to sit down if you have problems getting them to listen.
9	Use a whistle to attract attention rather than trying to shout over the top of the noise.
10	Frequent demonstrations have been shown to help children learn but make sure that your demonstrations are correct as well as frequent.
11	Verbal information has been shown to help visual demonstrations but limit the number of words used and the number of times feedback is given.
12	Information about errors has been shown to be more effective in improving skills than comments regarding correct actions.
13	Try to delay giving feedback until about 10 seconds after the skill practice.
14	Short and frequent sessions have been shown to be preferable for the improvement of gross motor skills so encourage children to practise as often as possible.
15	Always be positive and encourage children to have fun.

1. STEP THROUGHS

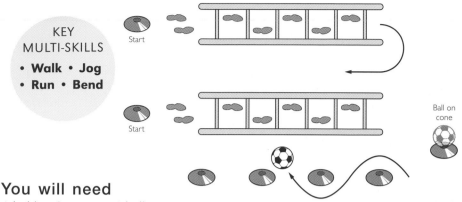

KEY
MULTI-SKILLS

- **Walk** • **Jog**
- **Run** • **Bend**

You will need

1 ladder, 6 x cones, 1 ball

START Walk through the ladder putting one foot in each square. At the end of the ladder turn and walk back to the start. The next person goes. Next, do this at a jog pace and then a faster pace.

TRY The first person steps through the ladder, picks up the ball, zig-zags back through the cones and passes the ball to the next person who runs through the ladder and places it back on the cone. Continue until each team member has had a go.

- -

2. SIDE STEPS

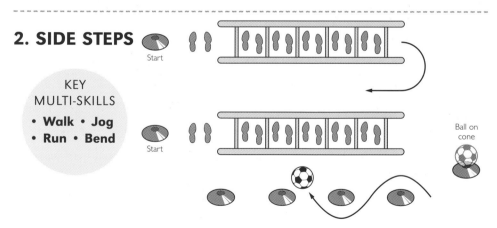

KEY
MULTI-SKILLS

- **Walk** • **Jog**
- **Run** • **Bend**

You will need

1 ladder, 6 x cones, 1 ball

START Walk sideways putting one foot in each rung of the ladder. At the end of the ladder turn and walk back to the start. The next person goes. Next, do this at a jog pace and then a faster pace.

TRY The first person sidesteps through the ladder, picks up the ball, zig-zags back through the cones and passes the ball to the next person who puts it back on the cone. Continue until each team member has had a go.

Movement skills with a ladder

3. SPOTTY DOG

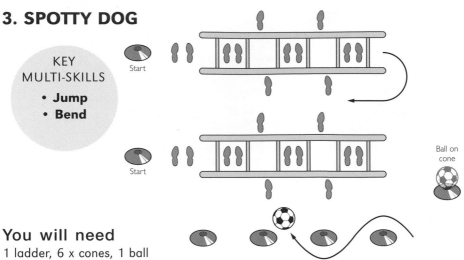

KEY
MULTI-SKILLS
• **Jump**
• **Bend**

You will need
1 ladder, 6 x cones, 1 ball

START Jump sideways into the first square of the ladder with both feet and then jump up and land with one foot in front of the next square and one foot behind (split stance). At the end of the ladder turn and walk back to the start. The next person goes. Next, do this at a jog pace and then a faster pace.

TRY The first person does spotty dog through the ladder, picks up the ball, zig-zags back through the cones and passes the ball to the next person who puts it back on the cone. Continue until each team member has had a go.

4. DOUBLE STEP THROUGHS

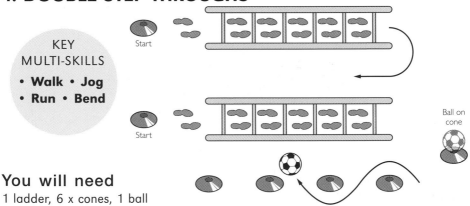

KEY
MULTI-SKILLS
• **Walk** • **Jog**
• **Run** • **Bend**

You will need
1 ladder, 6 x cones, 1 ball

START Walk through the ladder putting both feet in each square. At the end of the ladder turn and walk back to the start. The next person goes. Next, do this at a jog pace and then a faster pace.

TRY The first person does double step throughs along the ladder, picks up the ball, zig-zags back through the cones and passes the ball to the next person who puts it back on the cone. Continue until each team member has had a go.

5. LADDER TRAIN

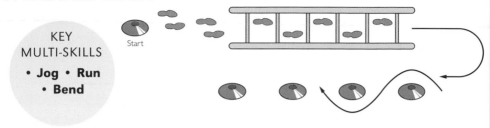

KEY
MULTI-SKILLS

• Jog • Run
• Bend

You will need
1 ladder, 5 x cones

START All of the group go through the ladders one after the other (at three-rung intervals) putting one foot in each square. At the end of the ladder the group zig-zag back through the cones.

TRY Different footwork from previous sessions.

---

6. DOUBLE HOPSCOTCH

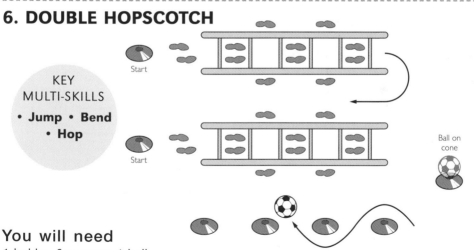

KEY
MULTI-SKILLS

• Jump • Bend
• Hop

You will need
1 ladder, 6 x cones, 1 ball

START Jump with two feet together into the first square of the ladder then jump with both feet outside of the next square (hopscotch). At the end of the ladder turn and walk back to the start. The next person goes. Next, do this at a jog pace and then a faster pace.

TRY First person does hopscotch along the ladder, picks up the ball, zig-zags back through the cones and passes the ball to the next person who puts it back on the cone. Continue until each team member has had a go.

199

7. SINGLE HOPSCOTCH

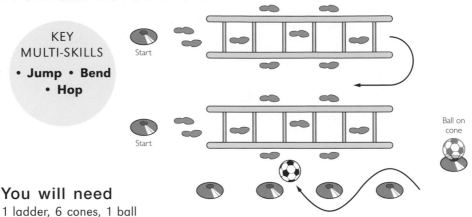

KEY
MULTI-SKILLS
• **Jump** • **Bend**
• **Hop**

Start

Start

Ball on
cone

You will need
1 ladder, 6 cones, 1 ball

START Jump on one foot into the first square and then jump with both feet outside of the next square (hopscotch). At the end of the ladder turn and walk back to the start. The next person goes. Next, do this at a jog pace and then a faster pace.

TRY The first person does double step throughs along the ladder, picks up the ball, zig-zags back through the cones and passes the ball to the next person who puts it back on the cone. Continue until each team member has had a go.

----

8. JUMP INS

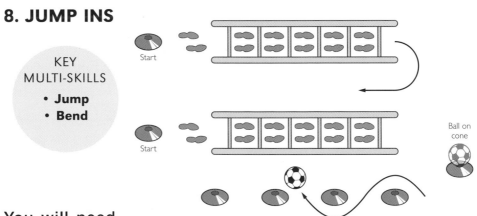

KEY
MULTI-SKILLS
• **Jump**
• **Bend**

Start

Start

Ball on
cone

You will need
1 ladder, 6 x cones, 1 ball

START Do two-footed jumps into each rung through the ladder. At the end of the ladder turn and walk back to the start. The next person goes. Next, do this at a jog pace and then a faster pace.

TRY The first person jumps along the ladder, picks up the ball, zig-zags back through the cones and passes the ball to the next person who puts it back on the cone. Continue until each team member has had a go.

9. HOP THROUGHS

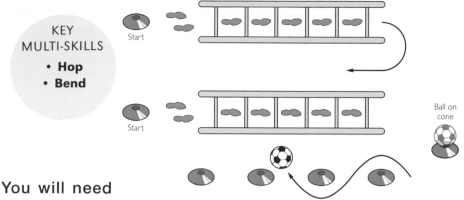

KEY MULTI-SKILLS

- **Hop**
- **Bend**

Start

Start

Ball on cone

You will need

1 ladder, 6 cones, 1 ball

START Hop on one foot into each square of the ladder. At the end of the ladder turn and walk back to the start. The next person goes. Next, do this at a jog pace and then a faster pace. Change legs.

TRY The first person hops along the ladder, picks up the ball, zig-zags back through the cones and passes the ball to the next person who puts it back on the cone. Continue until each team member has had a go.

- -

10. 3 AND 1

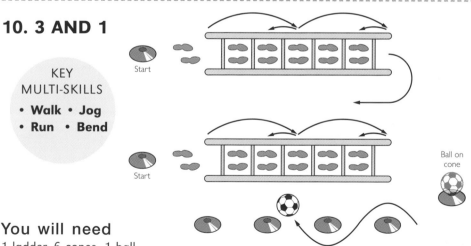

KEY MULTI-SKILLS

- **Walk** • **Jog**
- **Run** • **Bend**

Start

Start

Ball on cone

You will need

1 ladder, 6 cones, 1 ball

START Put one foot in each square of the ladder. After three squares, go back one square and then forward for three squares again. Repeat this all the way along the ladder. At the end of the ladder turn and walk back to the start. The next person goes.

TRY The first person does '3 and 1' through the ladder, picks up the ball, zig-zags back through the cones and passes the ball to the next person who puts it back on the cone. Continue until each team member has had a go.

Movement skills with a ladder

11. ZIG-ZAG

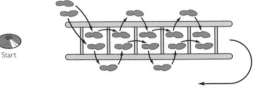
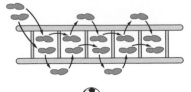

KEY
MULTI-SKILLS
• **Walk** • **Jog**
• **Run** • **Bend**

Start

Start

Ball on cone

You will need
1 ladder, 6 cones, 1 ball

START Stand slightly to the left side of the first square. Put the right foot in the first square followed by the left foot. Now put the right foot just outside (to the right) of the ladder and the left foot into the next square followed by the right foot. The left foot now goes outside of the ladder (to the left) and the right foot moves into the next square followed by the left, and so on.

TRY Start slowly and try to increase the pace. Use the ball and cones as in previous sessions.

12. ZIG AND RUN

KEY
MULTI-SKILLS
• **Walk** • **Jog**
• **Run** • **Bend**

Start

Start

Ball on cone

You will need
1 ladder, 6 cones, 1 ball

START As in activity 11, do the zig-zag for the first three squares in the ladder and then change to putting one foot in each of the remaining squares (run through). At the end of the ladder turn and walk back to the start. The next person goes.

TRY Start slowly and try to increase the pace. Use the ball and cones as in previous sessions.

1. STEP-OVERS

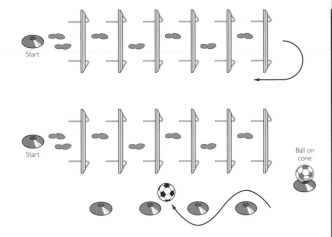

KEY
MULTI-SKILLS

- **Jump**
- **Bend**

You will need

6 x hurdles, 6 x cones, 1 ball

START Step over the middle of each hurdle but alternating the leading leg. At the end turn and walk back to the start. The next person goes. Next, do this at a jog pace and then a faster pace.

TRY The first person does step-overs on the hurdles, picks up the ball, zig-zags back through the cones and passes the ball to the next person who puts it back on the cone. Continue until each team member has had a go.

---

2. L-STEP-OVERS

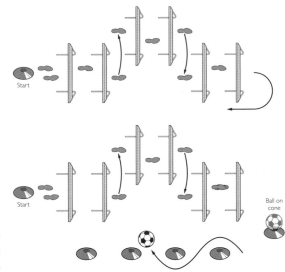

KEY
MULTI-SKILLS

- **Jump**
- **Bend**

You will need

6 x hurdles, 6 x cones, 1 ball

START Step over hurdles 1 and 2, but alternating the leading leg. Side-step to the left then step over 3 and 4. Side-step to the right and step over 5 and 6. At the end turn and walk back to the start. The next person goes. Next, do this at a jog pace and then a faster pace.

3. GALLOPS

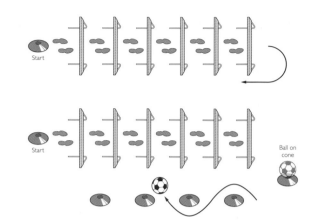

KEY
MULTI-SKILLS
- **Gallop**
- **Bend**

You will need

6 x hurdles, 6 x cones, 1 ball

START Step over each hurdle with the same leading leg. At the end turn and walk back to the start. The next person goes. Next, do this at a jog pace and then a faster pace. Repeat with the other leg leading.

TRY The first person does step-overs on the hurdles, picks up the ball, zig-zags back through the cones and passes the ball to the next person who puts it back on the cone. Continue until each team member has had a go.

- -

4. L-GALLOPS

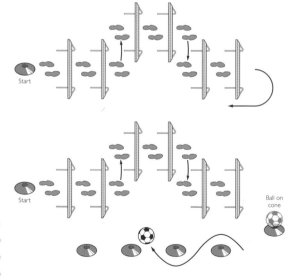

KEY
MULTI-SKILLS
- **Gallop**
- **Bend**

You will need

6 x hurdles, 6 x cones, 1 ball

START Step over hurdles 1 and 2 with the same leading leg. Side-step to the left then step over 3 and 4 with the same leg leading again. Side-step to the right and step over 5 and 6. At the end turn and walk back to the start. The next person goes. Next, do this at a jog pace and then a faster pace. Repeat with the other leg leading.

5. PEG LEG

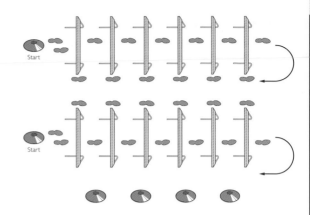

KEY
MULTI-SKILLS
• **Walk** • **Jog**
• **Run** • **Bend**

You will need
6 x hurdles, 5 x cones

START At walking pace, step over the edge of each hurdle with the left leg only by going down the right side of the hurdles. The right leg stays to the right side of the hurdle (like a peg leg). At the end, turn and walk back to the start. The next person goes. Next, do this at a jog pace and then a faster pace.

TRY Stepping over the hurdles with the right leg only (left leg to the side).

6. DOUBLE PEG LEG

KEY
MULTI-SKILLS
• **Walk** • **Jog**
• **Run** • **Bend**

You will need
6 x hurdles, 6 x cones

START Step over hurdle 1 and 2 with the
right leg only. Then step over 3 and 4 with the left leg only. Then step over 5 and 6 with the right leg again. At the end turn and walk back to the start. The next person goes. Next, do this at a jog pace and then a faster pace.

TRY Use more hurdles and change the order of the lead leg.

7. STAGGERED PEG LEG

KEY
MULTI-SKILLS
• **Walk** • **Jog**
• **Run**

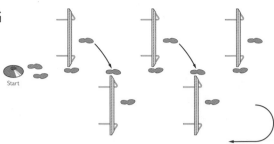

You will need
5 x hurdles, 1 cone

START Imagine a straight line up the middle so that hurdle 1 is just to the left of the line and hurdle 2 is just to the right, and so on. Peg leg over the right edge of hurdle 1 then over the left edge of hurdle 2 and so on. Start at walk pace and speed up. At the end turn and walk back to the start. Next person goes.

TRY Use more hurdles and change the order of the lead leg.

- -

8. PEG LEG HOP

KEY
MULTI-SKILLS
• **Walk** • **Jog**
• **Run**

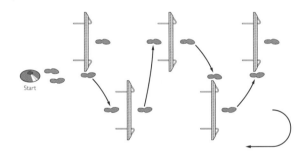

You will need
5 x hurdles, 1 cone

START Imagine a straight line up the middle so that hurdle 1 is just to the left of the line and hurdle 2 just to the right and so on. Peg leg over the right edge of hurdle 1 then hop over 2 with the right leg and hop over 3 with the left leg. Then peg leg over the left edge of hurdle 4 and repeat. At the end, turn and walk back to the start. The next person goes.

TRY Speeding up, but stay accurate.

9. SINGLE JUMPS

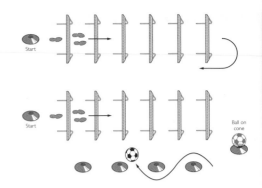

KEY MULTI-SKILLS

- **Jump**
- **Bend**

You will need
6 x hurdles, 6 x cones, 1 ball

START Jump over each hurdle (take off with one foot, land with two). At the end, turn and walk back to the start. The next person goes. Next, do this at a jog pace and then a faster pace.

TRY The first person jumps over the hurdles, picks up the ball, zig-zags back through the cones and passes the ball to the next person who puts it back on the cone. Continue until each team member has had a go.

---

10. SINGLE L-JUMPS

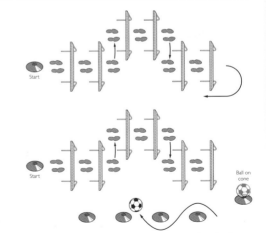

KEY MULTI-SKILLS

- **Jump**
- **Bend**

You will need
6 x hurdles, 6 x cones, 1 ball

START Jump over hurdles 1 and 2 taking off on one foot and landing with both feet. Side-step to the left then jump over 3 and 4. Side-step to the right and jump over 5 and 6. At the end, turn and walk back to the start. The next person goes. Next, do this at a jog pace and then a faster pace.

11. DOUBLE JUMPS

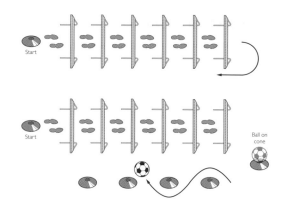

KEY
MULTI-SKILLS

• **Jump**
• **Bend**

You will need
6 x hurdles, 6 x cones, 1 ball

START Jump over each hurdle (take off and land with both feet). At the end turn and walk back to the start. The next person goes. Next, do this at a jog pace and then a faster pace.

TRY The first person jumps over the hurdles, picks up the ball, zig-zags back through the cones and passes the ball to the next person who puts it back on the cone. Continue until each team member has had a go.

----

12. DOUBLE L-JUMPS

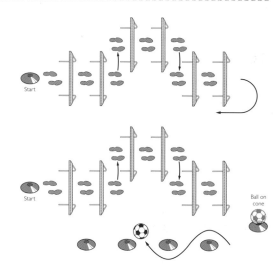

KEY
MULTI-SKILLS

• **Jump**
• **Bend**

You will need
6 x hurdles, 6 x cones, 1 ball

START Jump over hurdles 1 and 2 (take off and land with both feet). Side-step to the left then jump over 3 and 4. Side-step to the right and jump over 5 and 6. At the end, turn and walk back to the start. The next person goes. Next, do this at a jog pace and then a faster pace.

1. BALL BOUNCE

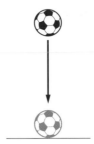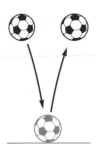

KEY
MULTI-SKILLS
• **Bounce**
• **Catch** • **Bend**

You will need
1 ball

START Bounce a ball on the floor as many times as possible with two hands. See how many times you can do this.

TRY Bouncing the ball with one hand then with the other hand. If successful, swap the bouncing hands without stopping.

- -

2. BOUNCE AND RUN

KEY
MULTI-SKILLS
• **Bounce**
• **Catch** • **Dribble**

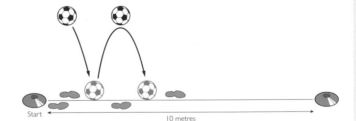

You will need
1 ball, 2 x cones

START Place two cones 10 metres apart. While bouncing a ball, run from one cone to the other and back again.

TRY Start using two hands to bounce and then use only one hand.

3. BOUNCE PASS

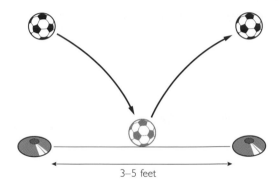

KEY
MULTI-SKILLS
• **Throw**
• **Catch** • **Sway**

3–5 feet

You will need
1 ball, 2 x cones

START In pairs, stand about 3–5 feet apart and bounce the ball to each other. The catcher must start by using two hands to catch the ball. Do not throw the ball too hard.

TRY Stand further apart. If successful, increase the speed of the throw.

---

4. BALL CATCH

KEY
MULTI-SKILLS
• **Throw**
• **Catch** • **Sway**

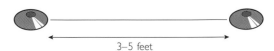

3–5 feet

You will need
1 ball, 2 x cones

START In pairs, stand about 3–5 feet apart and throw the ball to each other. The catcher must start by using two hands to catch the ball. Do not throw the ball too hard.

TRY Stand further apart. If successful, increase the speed of the throw.

5. BALL DRIBBLE

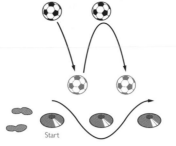

KEY
MULTI-SKILLS
- **Bounce**
- **Catch** • **Dribble**

You will need
1 ball, 6 x cones

START Bounce a ball and dribble through the cones and back to the start.

TRY Start using two hands to dribble and then use only one hand.

- -

6. HOOP ROLLS

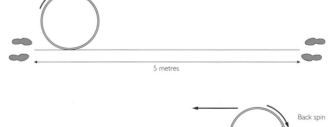

KEY
MULTI-SKILLS
- **Rotate**
- **Bend**

You will need
1 hoop

START In pairs, stand about 5 metres apart and roll the hoop along the floor to each other. Do not roll the hoop too fast.

TRY Use the left hand and then the right hand to roll the hoop. Try overhand and back spin, and/or standing further apart.

Manipulative skills with ball and hoop

7. HOOP TRAIN

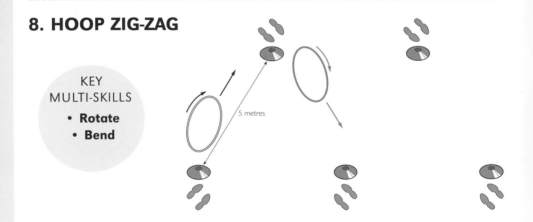

KEY
MULTI-SKILLS
- **Rotate**
- **Bend**

You will need
1 hoop

START Make a line. The first person rolls the hoop to the next person, who rolls to the next and so on, and then back again. When the hoop is back at the start, the person at the opposite end runs to the start position, takes the hoop and repeats.

TRY Use the left hand and then the right hand and then alternate in the same run.

8. HOOP ZIG-ZAG

KEY
MULTI-SKILLS
- **Rotate**
- **Bend**

5 metres

You will need
1 hoop, 5 x cones

START One person stands at each cone about 5 metres apart. Roll the hoop along the floor to the next person standing at each cone. Repeat this in the opposite direction.

TRY Use the left hand and then the right hand, both overhand and underhand.

9. GROUP HOOP

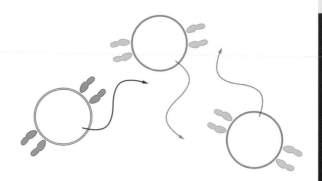

KEY
MULTI-SKILLS
• **Sway**
• **Run**

You will need
1 hoop

START In pairs rest the hoop against the tummy area and keep it up without using the hands. Walk around the room.

TRY In groups of four, each person will be touching a colour on the hoop. The coach calls out a colour. The person touching that colour on the hoop runs around the group and joins back in. The group have to keep the hoop up. Next, when a colour is called, the person touching that colour could run to join any other group, or when the coach shouts a colour, the person touching that colour could be given a task, i.e. touch all four corners of the room.

- -

10. HOOP SQUARE

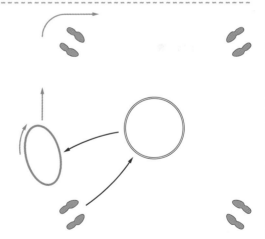

KEY
MULTI-SKILLS
• **Rotate**
• **Bend**

You will need
1 hoop

START Make a square around the hoop. The coach calls out a name. That person picks up the hoop and rolls it around the group and puts it back.

TRY Vary the shape of the group. Try rolling the hoop with one hand and two hands (forehand and backhand). Alternate the direction of the roll (clockwise and anti-clockwise).

213

Manipulative skills with ball and hoop

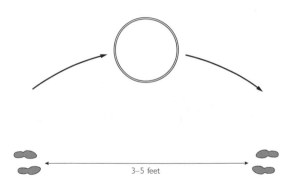

11. HOOP CATCH

KEY
MULTI-SKILLS
• **Throw**
• **Catch** • **Sway**

3–5 feet

You will need
1 hoop

START In pairs, stand about 3–5 feet apart and throw the hoop to each other. The catcher must start by using two hands to catch the hoop. Do not throw the hoop too high.

TRY Use the left hand and then the right hand to catch the hoop. Try standing further apart.

- -

12. COLOUR HOOP CATCH

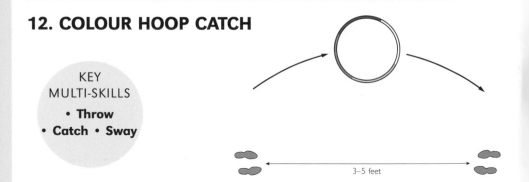

KEY
MULTI-SKILLS
• **Throw**
• **Catch** • **Sway**

3–5 feet

You will need
1 colour hoop

START In pairs, stand about 3–5 feet apart. Call out a colour and then throw the hoop to each other. The catcher must start by using two hands to catch the nominated colour on the hoop. Try not to spin the hoop too quickly.

TRY Use the left hand and then the right hand to catch the hoop. Try standing further apart. Spin the hoop a little more quickly. Hoops with coloured balls can also be used for this.

CHAPTER NINE

Health and safety

Objectives

After completing this chapter the reader should be able to:

- Describe the importance of screening and typical ways in which it is addressed.
- Define the term 'risk assessment' and describe common methods with typical examples.
- Describe what to do to give emergency first aid including contacting the emergency services.
- Understand the difference between minor and major injuries and how to use RICE for minor injuries.
- List and describe the areas related to child supervision, including coach-to-child ratio, hydration, environment and registers.
- Describe the procedure for accident or incident reporting.
- Explain the procedure for reporting any incidents under the child protection act.
- Describe different bullying situations and give advice on how to deal with them.
- Locate relevant codes of conduct.
- List the areas related to equal opportunities.
- List and describe the areas related to duty of care.

Introduction

It goes without saying that it is the responsibility of any children's coach to ensure the health and safety of all children (and of the coaches involved) while participating in any kind of coaching or physical activity or programme. It is important, therefore, that coaches are aware of all the health and safety policies relating to children and exercise and ensure that they are always strictly followed. It is also the responsibility of the coach to take action if there are any contraventions of any of the policies. Health and safety is a vast and ever-increasing area in which coaches must keep up to date. I have tried to address as many of the areas as possible that would come under the banner of health and safety such as:

- Screening
- Risk assessment
- Treatment of injuries
- First aid
- Contacting emergency services
- Emergency situations
- Supervision
- Accident or incident reporting
- Child protection
- Bullying
- Code of conduct
- Equal opportunities
- Duty of care

Screening

As with all exercise or activity delivery it is important to carry out a procedure known as 'screening' prior to the first session. Screening is simply the term used for checking as far as possible that there are no obvious health or fitness reasons that someone should not be participating in the activity. There are various levels of screening that can be done in order to help this process, as there are many types of pre-exercise health questionnaire (screening questionnaires) available. Unfortunately, most of the screening questionnaires that have been developed have been for adolescents and adults.

The most common and easy to use screening questionnaire is the Physical Activity Readiness Questionnaire (PAR-Q) as shown in figure 9.1, which was designed for those over the age of 15 years. This was developed by the Canadian Society for Exercise Physiology. The PAR-Q is a short questionnaire that can help to identify possible risk factors for cardiovascular, pulmonary and metabolic disease (in other words, is the individual at risk of certain diseases?). This screening process works very simply in that the questionnaire is given to an individual before they take part in any type of physical activity. If the individual answers 'yes' to any of the questions, then the form advises them to seek advice from their doctor before taking part in the activities. If the individual answers 'no' to all the questions, then it assumes that the individual is healthy enough to participate in any low- to moderate-intensity activities. The coach should note that the PAR-Q is a confidential document as it contains what is classed as sensitive information. For this reason, it should always be treated in a confidential manner and only be accessed by the coach.

Please read the following questions and answer each one honestly.

	Yes	No
1. Has your doctor ever said that you have a heart condition and that you should only do physical activity recommended by a doctor?	—	—
2. Do you feel pain in your chest when you do physical activity?	—	—
3. In the past month, have you had chest pain while you were not doing physical activity?	—	—
4. Do you lose your balance because of dizziness or do you ever lose consciousness?	—	—
5. Do you have a bone or joint problem that could be made worse by physical activity?	—	—
6. Is your doctor currently prescribing drugs for your blood pressure or heart condition?	—	—
7. Do you know of any other reason why you should not do physical activity?	—	—

If you answered YES to one or more questions

Talk to your doctor **BEFORE** you become more physically active or have a fitness appraisal. Discuss with your doctor which kinds of activities you wish to participate in.

If you answered NO to all questions

If you answered no to all questions you can be reasonably sure that you can:
- Start becoming much more physically active – start slow and build up.
- Take part in a fitness appraisal – this is a good way to determine your basic fitness level. It is recommended that you have your blood pressure evaluated.

However, delay becoming more active if:
- You are not feeling well because of temporary illness such as a cold or flu.
- If you are or maybe pregnant – talk to your doctor first.

Please note: *If your health changes so that you then answer YES to any of the above questions, tell your fitness or health professional. Ask whether you should change your physical activity plan.*

Fig. 9.1 Example of a PAR-Q questionnaire (reprinted with permission from the Canadian Society for Exercise Physiology). Continued overleaf

'I have read, understood and completed this questionnaire. Any questions I had were answered to my full satisfaction.'

Name_____

Signature_____   Date_____

Signature of parent_____   Witness_____
or guardian

Note: This physical activity clearance is valid for a maximum of 12 months from the date it is completed and becomes invalid if your condition changes so that you would answer YES to any of the seven questions.

Fig. 9.1 Continued

Screening for younger children (under 15 years of age) is different from that for adults as there is not a commonly accepted process or questionnaire that could be used. As guidance is somewhat limited in this area, many centres and clubs tend to use their own templates even though the validity and indeed the legality of the content would in many cases be contested. One possible reason for doing this could be to show that as a coach (or centre, club etc.) all possible measures were taken to ensure that children appeared healthy enough to take part in physical activity and there was no apparent reason why they shouldn't.

Fortunately there are very few health incidents that occur as a result of children taking part in physical activity but regardless of this, a simple screening process for younger children is always recommended not only from a legal perspective but also in trying to identify those children that might require special attention. Figure 9.2 is an example of one of many screening templates for children that could be used. These questionnaires tend to be called 'readiness questionnaires'.

Fig. 9.2 Example of a readiness questionnaire for children

Readiness Questionnaire for Children

Dear parent or guardian, please could you complete the following form. Even though, for most children, physical activity is very beneficial, there are a small number of children who may be at risk when participating in a physical activity programme. Your child cannot participate in any such activity programme until this form has been completed and reviewed by the coach. Please note that the information contained in this form is confidential.

Personal child details

Name: .... DOB: .... M/F: ....

Height: .... Weight: ....

Name of parent(s) or guardian(s): ....

Home address:

....

....

.... Post code: ....

Contact numbers: ....

Emergency contact name: .... Contact number: ....

Relationship to child: ....

- -

Has your child got or ever had: Y   N

A heart condition (please specify) .... ☐ ☐

Diabetes (type 1 or 2 - please specify) .... ☐ ☐

Cystic fibrosis .... ☐ ☐

High blood pressure .... ☐ ☐

High cholesterol .... ☐ ☐

Breathing problems or shortness of breath (e.g. asthma) .... ☐ ☐

Continued

Epilepsy or seizures/convulsions .... ☐ ☐
If yes, is it at rest or during exercise? ....

Fainting or dizzy spells .... ☐ ☐

Increased bleeding / haemophilia .... ☐ ☐

If your child is taking any medication, please list and state if there are any side effects experienced as a result of taking this medication:
....

	Y	N

Has your child ever broken any bones?................................. ☐ ☐
If yes, what bones and when?...

Does your child have any muscular pain while exercising?...................... ☐ ☐
If yes, explain where and what the pain is:
....

Does your child experience any joint pains? .... ☐ ☐
If yes, explain where and what the pain is:
....

Does your child suffer from any allergies?.. ☐ ☐
If yes, please list allergies and any special requirements:
....

Does your child have cerebral palsy?.. ☐ ☐

Does your child have ADHD?.. ☐ ☐

Are you aware of any medical condition or other reason that might prevent your child from participating in an exercise programme?......... ☐ ☐
If yes, please explain:
....

I hereby acknowledge that:

The information provided above regarding my child's health is, to the best of my knowledge, correct and I will inform you immediately if there are any changes to the information provided above.

I give permission for my child to participate in your activity programme.

Name of parent/guardian (block caps): ....

Parent/guardian signature: ....   Date:..............

Approved for participation (block caps): ....

Signature: ....   Date:..............

Fig. 9.2 Example of a readiness questionnaire for children

You will see from the example questionnaire in figure 9.2 that there is much more information relating to health than the PAR-Q for over 15s. There is a lot more information that could be asked relating to the health of the child but if this is done, completing the form then becomes laborious and unrealistic for the parents. The example covers many areas relating to childhood conditions but if the coach feels that they need more information then it is at their discretion. Coaches could ask for information relating to exercise history but this could also be done in a goal setting session (*see* chapter 7).

Once the readiness questionnaire has been completed it is up to the coach to deal with any issues reported. As many of the issues are medically-related, it is suggested that if in doubt, the coach refers the issue to the child's doctor for approval to take part in the activity programme with any exercise conditions that the coach needs to be aware of, such as limiting the intensity or the duration of the exercise.

Readiness questionnaires are not the only type of screening that should be carried out for children as injury screening is also another important area that the coach should be aware of. It is often the case that a child turns up to an activity session with an acute (recently happened) injury that had occurred after they had completed either a PAR-Q questionnaire or another type of screening questionnaire. If this does happen, then whether or not the child takes part in the session should be discussed with the parent or guardian (prior to them joining in with the session). If the parents or guardians are not available at the time to discuss this then the nature of the acute injury should be assessed as best as possible and if the coach deems the child is unfit to continue, then the parent or guardian should be contacted and the child should not be allowed to take part in the session (for their own good). It is important, therefore, that even if screening forms (whichever are being used) have been completed by all the children taking part in a particular activity programme, it is a good habit to ask all the children prior to the start of each session if they have any current injuries or illnesses that they may not have had when they first completed the screening forms. In other words, are they injured at the time? This kind of check done at the start of all activity sessions is known as 'verbal screening'.

Risk assessment

In any form of exercise or physical activity, there are associated risks or situations that might occur not only to the participants but to the coaches as well. Although it is difficult to eradicate all risks completely (as playing any sport or activity has risks), it is important to recognise the potential risks, and plan to minimise them if possible. When planning an activity session, it is wise to carry out (and document) a risk assessment. This simply means thinking about any possible risks that there might be and how to try to deal with them to make them less of a risk. Often a good place to start is by asking questions about the activity that you are going to do. Table 9.1 helps you to do this by giving a typical scenario response to general risk questions.

Table 9.1 Risk assessment questions

Question	Scenario response
1 Are there any potential hazards which might result in significant harm?	The use of foot ladders could result in tripping and injury caused by falling.
2 Who might be harmed?	The coach or the participants.
3 Is the risk of significant harm low/unlikely, medium/possible or high/probable?	Medium.
4 Where the risk is identified as medium or high, has an action been identified?	Only use the ladders on grass to lessen the impact on falling. Only allow one person at a time on the ladder.

Each question would then need a risk rating of low, medium or high. What actually constitutes a low-, medium- or high-risk situation might be slightly different depending on how each individual coach perceives each situation. Whatever the coach's perception of the rating of a situation within an activity session, the following guidelines could be applied:

- Low risk: Further precautions are optional and the activity can go ahead
- Medium risk: Further precautions should be taken before the activity proceeds
- High risk: The risk should be reduced before running the activity

If there are medium or high risks associated with the session then a risk assessment must be carried out. There are many types of risk assessment form that can be used but the template in figure 9.3 (partially filled in with example risks) can be used to help formulate and document a basic risk assessment.

Risk Assessment Form

Venue:............................... Date of check: ....

Session leader: .... Session: Circuit and weights

Potential Risk	Lo Med Hi	Method of minimising risk	Action to be taken
Participant recovering from shoulder injury	Med	Limit range of motion and weight	Set pec dec range to start at limited range of motion
Participants could run into walls in indoor venue	Med	Limit running area	Use cones to set the limits of the session away from the walls
Participants might have to wait if machines busy	Lo	Give alternative exercise	Have cards with alternatives for this scenario

                                                                           Y   N

Register .... ☐ ☐

Suitable clothing .... ☐ ☐

Fig. 9.3 Example of a typical risk assessment form (continued on page 224)

Emergency points .... ☐ ☐

First-aid kit .... ☐ ☐

Telephone .... ☐ ☐

Water .... ☐ ☐

Signed: ....   Date: ....

Name: ....

Fig. 9.3 Continued

Treatment of injuries

It is very common that injuries occur during activity sessions, especially with children. Depending on the nature of the injury, treatment may be given on site at the time it happens if the injury is not serious (known as a 'minor injury'). If, however, the injury is of a more serious nature (known as a 'major injury'), the injured child may require some sort of outside medical attention. It is not possible to list all the possible minor and major injuries but the coach could use the following list as a guide. For more detailed information relating to minor and major injury treatment, it is recommended to use one of many available first-aid books.

- Minor injuries: These types of injury can be given treatment on site – injuries such as cuts and bruises.
- Major injuries: These types of injury require outside medical attention – fainting, asthma, overexertion, heat exhaustion, sprains and strains, diabetic emergency, epilepsy and heart failure.

Under the heading of major injuries, sprains and strains are also known as 'soft-tissue' injuries as they are injuries caused to either muscle, tendon or ligament (soft) tissue. Even though these types of injury require specialist people (such as physiotherapists) to deal with them, the coach can still give immediate treatment to a child with a soft-tissue injury as it will help until they can be taken to the specialist for further treatment. The immediate treatment that the coach can provide for all injuries such as these is known by the acronym RICE. This treatment in simple terms is done in order to reduce the amount of swelling at the site of the injury. Figure 9.4 shows the RICE treatment that can be given.

R	Rest	Rest, steady and support the injured part of the body.
I	Ice	Apply an ice pack or cold compress. This will reduce swelling and pain.
C	Compress	Apply gentle compression to help reduce swelling.
E	Elevate	Raise the injured part to reduce blood flow to the area.

Fig. 9.4 RICE procedures

First aid

Every organisation (club, sports centre etc.) should have their own first-aid policy and reporting procedure that is made available for all coaches. It would be wise for coaches to have a copy of this and make themselves familiar with it. Coaches should also ensure that there is a qualified first-aider at the venue whenever they are coaching but it would be better if the coach had some sort of first-aid training themselves. Coaches should always make sure that they have information on every child's individual medical background and any injuries, and they should pay particular attention to any allergies (anaphylactic shock, plasters) that they have been told about. It is also the responsibility of the coach to make sure that a first-aid kit is available at all sessions. This kit should be maintained at all times and should never contain any pills or creams. During any activity session it is possible that the coach may have to deal with an emergency situation which is why it is always better if coaches are trained in emergency first aid. If an emergency does occur that requires first aid, the same procedure should always be followed.

Emergency aid procedure

1 Assess the situation. Approach quickly but remain calm. Identify any risks to yourself, the casualties and bystanders.
2 If you judge the situation to be life threatening call the emergency services immediately.
3 Make the area safe. The conditions that caused the emergency may still be a problem.
4 Give emergency aid. Assess the casualty and give any necessary first aid.
5 Get help. Send someone for help or telephone for assistance.
6 Comfort the casualty. Reassure the casualty until help arrives.
7 Keep the casualty warm and comfortable.

Contacting emergency services

When a coach or a resident first-aider gives emergency aid, it is often the case that the emergency services (usually an ambulance) are then required. Sometimes the coach is a bit reluctant or unsure whether to call the emergency services or not but it is always better to be safe than sorry. You could always explain the incident to the emergency services who will then offer advice on whether or not they are needed. If the situation does arise, when calling the emergency services it is important that they are given the full information and details regarding the nature of the incident. It is important to remember however, that when calling the emergency services the 'control room' or the operator that you speak to may not be local: therefore you will have to explain things in detail. For instance, you might need to fully describe such things as the location and whereabouts of the incident because the operator you are talking to will not be familiar with where you are. If you do need to call the emergency services then the following procedure would be useful.

Contacting emergency services procedure

1 Keep calm and speak clearly.
2 Give your full name and state which service you require.
3 Give the full name, address and telephone number of the club or facility where the session is being held.
4 Give the exact location details and time of the accident/incident.
5 Give the number and condition of any casualties and details of any treatment which is being or has been given.
6 Give the access point for the ambulance.
7 Instruct someone to meet the ambulance, which will help them to reach the casualty as quickly as possible.

Emergency situations

A coach may also find themselves in the situation where they have to deal with emergency procedures such as fires, security incidents or missing persons. When dealing with an emergency it is important that the coach follows the emergency operating procedures (EOPs) that are available from all places of work (if they are not available then ask for them as they are a legal requirement). The coach will need to familiarise themselves with the EOPs at each site that they work from as they will be different. As a simple guideline the following procedure can be adhered to during an emergency situation.

Emergency operating procedure

1 Inform people involved about correct emergency procedures.
2 Follow procedures in a calm but correct manner.

3 Maintain the safety of those involved at all times.

4 Clearly and accurately report any problems to a responsible colleague.

5 Make a detailed report of the incident afterwards.

Supervision

There are several common areas that come under the heading of supervision (such as coach-to-child ratio, environment, hydration and register) that can be discussed briefly.

Coach-to-child ratio

As there are no legal requirements for the number of coaches required to supervise a certain number of children, this is left to the discretion of the coach. In a group activity scenario I would recommend that there should be no more than 20 children to each coach. Applying this maximum ratio is important for many reasons such as being able to physically see the entire group taking part in order to identify any potential danger as quickly as possible. The Office for Standards in Education (OFSTED) do however publish guidelines on coach-to-child ratios for younger children, as shown in table 9.2.

Table 9.2 OFSTED guidelines for coach-to-child supervision

Age (years)	Coach/child ratio
Under 2	1:3
2–3	1:4
3–7	1:8

Environment

There are many guidelines relating to the environment. The American body the National Association for Sport and Physical Education (NASPE) are quite comprehensive in their recommendations, which are summarised as follows:

- A space of at least 5 feet (1.5m) by 7 feet (2.1m) for each child should be allowed for structured movement (this is quite a large space).
- All surfaces should be clear of obstructions, dirt and sharp objects.
- Sharp objects and small parts to toys or games should be out of reach.
- Risk assessment of every venue must be carried out.

- Health disclosures from parents must be provided.
- If the temperature exceeds 30°C (86°F), children should not exercise for longer than 20 minutes and should be well hydrated before, during and after exercise.
- If the temperature exceeds 38°C (100°F), children should not exercise outside.

Hydration

It is important for all children (and adults) to drink water before, during and after exercise as fluids are continually being lost as a result of sweating and breathing and must be replaced. Children have a higher percentage of body water than adults, and therefore lose more fluid during exercise. Children also have a less efficient cooling system than adults and tend to heat up faster: they are also susceptible to overheating. For more information on children and hydration, see chapter 4.

Register

Before all sessions it is important that coaches complete a register of *all* the children and ensure that relevant children have any medication they have been prescribed (these details should have been collected before the start of the activity programme). Coaches can make up their own templates for registers as these should be simple documents with brief information relating to the venue, the date and the names of all the children who have attended the session (even if they did not take part for some reason they still need to be registered and supervised).

Accident or incident reporting

In the event of an accident or an incident occurring during an activity session in which the coach is in charge, an accident/incident report must be completed as a record of the event for future use if necessary. The coach should note that it is a legal requirement to immediately report all accidents and occurrence of dangerous incidents. The centre from which the coach is working must provide the form or booklet for the coach to make this report.

As well as being a legal requirement to complete a report, it should also be noted that there is a statutory requirement to keep accident records for a period of at least three years.

Child protection

The Protection of Children Act 1999 was designed to increase the level of protection for children by screening those wishing to supervise children in order to identify those not suitable to do so. Those deemed unsuitable would be people on the following lists:

- List 99 from The Department for Education And Skills (DfES)
- Department of Health list
- National Assembly of Wales list

Note: National governing bodies are required to have child protection policies. Clubs and organisations should also have a child protection policy and designated liaison. Local authorities provide policies and expertise and social services offer a wide range of support. For more information regarding policies go to: www.sportprotects.org.uk. Anyone wishing to deliver children's activities is required to carry out a disclosure check which cross-references lists such as those above. It is common that the environment in which coaches work will have in place the procedures required for the disclosure check. If you require more information on this process you should visit the following website: www.disclosure.gov.uk. Most coaches think that child protection is an area that doesn't concern them but it is crucial to protect the coach and the child from any potentially difficult situations. Physical contact with children should always be kept to a minimum regardless of the situation. There are, however, situations where contact cannot be avoided. For example:

- Demonstrating the use of certain equipment
- Helping to tie shoelaces
- Providing a steadying hand during gymnastic type movements

In these situations it is important that the coach maintains a professional, non-sexual approach. There are also situations that often arise where a child requires help and, although the intention may be innocent, could be perceived wrongly by others, for example helping a child to get changed. In these situations, coaches should find an alternative method such as asking one of the other children to help. Above all, the golden rule for coaches is *never* be left in a one-to-one situation with any child. If a situation arises where the last child is waiting for parents and you are the only coach present, wait in an area where other people are around (for example in the reception area of the club in which you are coaching).

For those who are frequently involved in coaching, there may be a situation in which a child approaches you and divulges sensitive information about potential abuse by another coach or adult. Even though this puts you in a very delicate situation, it is not your responsibility to decide if child abuse or inappropriate behaviour has taken place, so you must report the incident immediately. If you are working on behalf of a company then your report should go to head office. If you are a self-employed coach then you need to report to the governing body of the sport that you are coaching. You can use a simple form such as the example in figure 9.5 to make your report (*see* the following sections for more details on what to report).

Child Protection – Incident Report Form

Name of child ....

Age ....   Date of Birth ....

Address ....

....   Postcode ....

What happened (in child's own words if possible)

....

....

....

When the incident happened ....

Where the incident happened ....

When was the incident reported ....

Coach's observations (i.e. description of behaviour or injury)

....

....

....

Name of coach (block caps) ....

Signed ....   Date

Fig. 9.5 Example of a child protection incident report form

Bullying

Bullying is not as straightforward as it might first appear, because there are various forms of bullying. Verbal bullying and physical bullying (these terms are self-explanatory) are just two of the forms, but whatever the nature of the bullying it is very unpleasant and should be reported or dealt with immediately. That said, it is important that coaches should assess any potential bullying situation carefully if, and before, any action is taken. In some cases when verbal abuse occurs between children (by either party), it is often enough for the coach to give out warnings to the children concerned to hopefully prevent any further incidents occurring. If the verbal abuse continues, then punishment such as a 'time-out' could be given to those children involved.

Definition

A 'time-out' just means taking the child out of the activity for a few minutes.

If the time-out doesn't work and the verbal abuse continues, then the children responsible should be removed from the remainder of the session. Physical abuse between children should also be dealt with immediately. In most cases a 'time-out' would be appropriate and suffice followed by removal from the session if the physical abuse continues. If the physical abuse continues into following sessions, then it may be necessary to report the incidents to a parent.

Did you know

Eight out of ten children in the UK report being bullied on a regular basis.

It is also sometimes the case that a parent mentions that their son or daughter is being 'picked on' during a coaching session you are taking. If they do this it is possible that you might not be aware of it. If this is the case then you may agree with the parent to observe the situation over future sessions and report back to the parent. It is common that parents want to do this confidentially without the knowledge of the child: as a coach you must respect this choice.

Coaches should be aware that reports of 'bullying' are very common but can some-times be fabricated for the purpose of attention-seeking, especially by younger children. For this reason, coaches should only ever deal with what they directly observe as opposed to hearsay. This is not to say that the complaint should be ignored, and so the coach should observe future sessions with particular attention. If coaches feel uncomfortable dealing with, or making a report of, any incident, senior coaches should be contacted as soon as possible for advice.

Code of conduct

Most professions will make available codes of conduct for those who are working within them. Codes of conduct in this case give deliverers practical information relevant to the coaching of young children. Codes of conduct can be found covering both sport for coaches and also health and fitness for exercise instructors.

- For sport: Code of Practice for Sports Coaches – available from www.1st4sport.com
- For health and fitness: Code of Conduct – available from www.skillsactive.co.uk

Equal opportunities

The term 'equal opportunities' simply relates to making sure that opportunities to take part in a sport or activity are the same for everyone regardless of race, colour, creed or religion etc. It is actually the responsibility of the coach to ensure that each session that they deliver is fair, open and accessible to everyone who wants to take part. Coaches are obliged to do this as Government legislation dictates that it is a legal requirement to provide equal opportunities for everyone in all sporting events that they are involved in. The following statement relating to equal opportunities was made by Sport England in 2000:

> Sports equity is about fairness in sport, equality of access, recognising inequalities and taking steps to address them. It is about changing the culture and structure of sport to ensure that it becomes equally accessible to everyone in society.

The extent of information relating to equal opportunities is extensive, and therefore organisations such as The National Coaching Foundation and Sportscoach UK have proposed the acronym RAFT to help coaches identify and understand their responsibilities in this area, as shown in Table 9.3.

Table 9.3 RAFT for equal opportunities		
R	Recognising inequalities	Coaches need to acknowledge that certain groups are under-represented in all areas of sport.
A	Access	Coaches need to provide sporting opportunities for everyone within the context of their ability and activity.
F	Fairness	Coaches must treat all participants equally, but be aware that some people may need more support than others. Coaches must recognise that different people have different needs and aspirations.
T	Taking action	Coaches must take positive action to ensure that their sport becomes equally accessible to everyone in society.

Duty of care

According to Her Majesty's Government, any adult who works with children has something known as a 'duty of care'. This means that those working with children have a responsibility to keep children safe and protect them from sexual, physical and emotional harm. Failure to do this could be regarded as neglect and could lead to prosecution. For full details regarding duty of care, coaches should go to the website www.everychildmatters.gov.uk or purchase a copy of 'Working Together to Safeguard Children: 2006 HM Government'. For the purpose of this book we will look briefly at the areas of duty of care concerned with coaching children which are summarised in table 9.4.

Confidentiality

Coaches often have information about their players that is confidential (address, contact details etc.) which means that the information must be treated as such at all times. If a coach is not sure about what information is confidential or how to treat it, they should access a copy of the Data Protection Act 1998, which provides all the information relevant to this area.

Sexual conduct

The Sexual Offences Act 2003 in relation to abuse of positions of trust states that, where a person aged 18 years of age or over is in a specified position of trust with a child under 18 years of age, it is an offence for that person to engage in sexual activity with or in the presence of that child, or to cause or incite that child to engage in or watch sexual activity. There is absolutely no ambiguity about this statement as it means any sexual activity is a criminal offence! It does happen quite often, though, that children become infatuated with their coaches. This is a very sensitive situation in which coaches must be highly professional at all times and if a coach does suspect some kind of infatuation they must speak with a senior person immediately. Coaches should be especially aware that showing special attention to certain children, regardless of their gender, can sometimes be seen by others as 'grooming'.

Social contact

In simple terms, coaches should not seek to have social contact with players or their families. In practice however, this is not always easy as many coaches already have social contact with families before undertaking a coaching role. Even if this is the case, coaches should never allow players in their own home without the presence of their parents. In circumstances like this, the coach should be as professional as possible at all times and keep managers or supervisors aware of the situation.

Communication

This area relates to the use of mobile phones, emails, websites, cameras, videos etc. Coaches should always be mindful of anything that could be construed as grooming. For instance, personal mobile or home numbers should never be given out and any communication using mediums such as social networking sites should never be used. Any communication either to or from the coach should always be done through the parent or guardian. This also applies if the coach is wanting to video or take pictures of the players for reasons such as improving technique or analysing game situations. Written permission from the parents of *all* children must be collected before the event.

Physical contact

This is probably an area that frightens all coaches as in many situations physical contact with players is necessary from a coaching perspective. Children can feel really uncomfortable with physical contact, so the coach should always ask the child if it is alright to do this and explain the purpose and what they are going to do. For instance, the grip of a racquet might need to be adjusted so the coach will need to make contact with the hand and wrist of the player in order to do so. Coaches should be professional in the way they do this and never appear to be secretive or make lingering contact in any way.

It is often good practice to inform parents of what you are doing (especially for very young children) so they understand the need for the contact. Unfortunately it is sometimes the case that children who have suffered abuse may seek inappropriate contact with the coach. Whether or not this is the case, any situation where a child initiates inappropriate contact should be dealt with. The coach needs to make the boundaries clear to the child (in a sensitive way) but then report the matter to a senior person as soon as possible.

Comforting

I don't think there is a coach who has never had the instance of a child who has become upset for some reason or another. Our instincts to put an arm around the shoulder for the purpose of comfort can be very strong but we should always think twice in these situations, especially when working one-to-one with a child. The coach should use their professional judgement in each case as the circumstances could be very different. For instance, a child might become upset because they didn't perform well, so a reassuring hand on the shoulder or pat on the back would be enough in this case. In the case of a young child falling and hurting themselves, an arm around the shoulder might be needed to console the child if they are in a state of distress. The coach should be aware of any child trying to feign distress in order to gain sympathy. In any case which the coach feels unsure about they should record the incident and the nature of what happened.

Care

Depending on the age of the child, problems related to areas such as changing and bathing can occur. It is good practice for the coach to organise this right at the beginning to avoid any such problems. You might agree with the parents that the child already comes and leaves in their training kit; however, they might need to change into strips for match purposes. A coach should always check that all children are changed before going into a changing facility for team talks and so on (do not enter a changing room with children of the opposite gender). If a particular child has a problem changing or bathing then allocate one of their friends to help them. It may also be the case that you have to assist children with disabilities. Always check with the parents first and establish procedures for care.

Table 9.4 Summary of the duty of care areas

Area	Main points	Advice	Information
Confidentiality	● Treat all information about players as confidential ● Do not allow others access to this information	● Keep confidential information in a lockable place	● Data Protection Act 1998
Sexual conduct	● All sexual activity is a criminal offence ● Special attention can be construed as grooming	● Never make sexual remarks or jokes ● Never discuss your own relationship	● Sexual Offences Act 2003 ● Working Together to Safeguard Children: 2006

Area	Main points	Advice	Information
	• Report any concerns about infatuation	• Always make contact by email or phone through the parent or guardian • Avoid having favourites and giving special attention	• HM Government
Social contact	• Social contact between coaches and players is not encouraged • Coaches should not invite players to their homes or use them to do errands	• Make supervisors aware of any social contact with players and their families. • Never allow players into your home without their parents	
Communication	• Communication includes phones, emails, websites and cameras • Contact is only needed in professional instances such as informing that sessions are cancelled	• Always communicate through the parent or guardian • Always get written permission for photos or videos	
Physical contact	• Physical contact is often required in coaching as long as it is appropriate • Some children may feel uncomfortable by this whereas others may initiate inappropriate contact	• Get permission from children before any contact • Try to keep parents informed of the need for this contact in coaching	• Most sports' governing body policies

Area	Main points	Advice	Information
	● There may be cultural or religious issues	● Make sure children know of the boundaries ● Report any issues immediately	
Comforting	● Children often become distressed for many reasons, especially younger children ● Some children may use this to seek comfort ● Professional judgement is key	● Often a hand on the shoulder is enough to comfort ● Never comfort in a one-to-one situation unless another coach or parent is present ● Record any issues you may be unsure about	
Care	● This relates to changing, bathing and toileting ● It may also relate to children with specific disabilities	● Check with parents about any toilet issues ● Ask the child if they would like help from one of their friends ● If in doubt, check with parents and establish ground rules	● Professional codes of practice

Bibliography

American College of Sports Medicine (ACSM) (2006). *ACSM's Guidelines for Exercise Testing and Prescription* (7th edn). Baltimore, Maryland, Lea & Febiger

Andren-Sandberg, A. (1998). 'Athletic training of children and adolescents: Growth and maturation more important than training for endurance in the young'. *Lakartidningen*, 95(41):4480–4487

Annual Report of the Chief Medical Officer (2000). 'Obesity – Defusing the health time-bomb'. Health Check, 37–45

Armstrong, N., Williams, J., Balding, J., Gentle, P. and Kirby, B. (1991). 'Cardiopulmonary fitness, physical activity patterns, and selected coronary risk factor variables in 11 to 16 year olds'. *Pediatric Exercise Science*, 3:219–228

Armstrong, N., McManus, A., Welsman, J. and Kirby, B. (1996). 'Physical activity patterns and aerobic fitness among prepubescents'. *European Physical Education Review*, 2(1):19–29

Armstrong, N. and Welsman, J. (1997). *Young People and Physical Activity*. Oxford, Oxford University Press

Aronne, L.J. (2002). 'Classification of obesity and assessment of obesity related health risks'. *Obesity Research*, 10:105S–115S

Aruajo, T., Matsudo, S., Andrade, D., Matsudo, V., Andrade, R., Rocha, A., Andrade, E. and Rocha, J. (1997). 'Physical fitness and physical activity levels of schoolchildren'. In J. Welsman, N. Armstrong and B. Kirby (eds.), *Children and Exercise Volume II*. XIXth International Symposium of Pediatric Work Physiology, Exeter, UK, 1997. Exeter, Washington Singer Press, 91–96

Avon Longitudinal Study of Parents and Children (1998). Health Survey for England 2001

Baquet, G., Berthoin, S., Dupont, G., Blondel, N., Fabre, C. and Van Praagh, E. (2002). 'Effects of high intensity intermittent training on peak VO_2 in prepubertal children'. *International Journal of Sports Medicine*, 06:439–444

Baquet, G., Berthoin, S., Gerbeaux, M. and Van Praagh, E. (2001). 'High-intensity aerobic training during a 10 week one-hour physical education cycle: Effects on physical fitness of adolescents aged 11 to 16'. *International Journal of Sports Medicine*, 04:295–300

Barlow, S. and Dietz, W.H. (1998). 'Obesity evaluation and treatment: Expert committee recommendations'. *Pediatrics*, 102(3):e29

Bar-Or, O. (1993). 'Physical activity and physical training in childhood obesity'. *Journal of Sports Medicine and Physical Fitness*, 33:323-329

Bar-Or, O. and Baronowski, T. (1994). 'Physical activity, adiposity and obesity among adolescents'. *Pediatric Exercise Science*, 6:348-360

Bayli, I. (1999). *A Parents/Coaches Guide: Developing the Young Soccer Player, Ages 6 to 21*. Lincoln, Nebraska, Performance Conditioning Inc.

Bayli, I. (2001). 'Keys to Success: Long Term Athlete Development'. Society of Weight Training Injury Symposium, Canada

Biddle, S., Sallis, J. and Cavill, N. (1998). 'Young and Active? Young People and Health Enhancing Physical Activity – Evidence and Implications'. London, Health Education Authority

Bompa, T.O. (1999). *Periodization: Theory and Methodology of Training* (4th edn). Champaign, Illinois, Human Kinetics

Bompa, T.O. (2000). *Total Training for Young Champions*. Champaign, Illinois, Human Kinetics

Boreham, C. and Riddoch, C. (2004). 'The physical activity, fitness and health of children'. *Journal of Sports Sciences*, 19(12):915-929

Borms, J. (1986). 'The child and exercise: An overview'. *Journal of Sports Science*, 4(1):3-20

Bouchard, C., Shephard, R.J., Stephens, T., Sutton, J.R. and McPherson, B.D. (1990) *Exercise, Fitness and Health: A consensus of current knowledge*. Champaign, Illinois, Human Kinetics

Braet, C., Mervielde, I. and Vandereycken, W. (1997). 'Psychological aspects of childhood obesity: A controlled study in a clinical and non-clinical sample'. *Journal of Paediatric Psychology*, 22(1):59-71

The British Association of Sport and Exercise Sciences Guide (2006) *Sport and Exercise Physiology Testing Guidelines*, ed. Jones, Andrew M., Winter, Edward M., Richard Davison, R.C., Bromley, Paul D., Mercer, Tom. Kentucky, USA, Routledge

British Heart Foundation (BHF) (2003). *Coronary Heart Disease Statistics – British Heart Foundation Statistics Database 2003*. London, BHF

British Medical Association (BMA) (2005). *Preventing Childhood Obesity*. London, BMA Publishing Unit

Brownell, K.D., Kelman, J.H. and Stunkard, A.J. (1983). 'Treatment of obese children with and without their mothers: Changes in weight and blood pressure'. *Pediatrics*, 71:515-23

Bundred, P., Kitchener, D. and Buchan, I. (2001). 'Prevalence of overweight and obese children between 1989 and 1998: Population based series of cross sectional studies'. *British Medical Journal*, 322:326-8

Burke, G.L., Jacobs, D.R., Sprafka, J.M., Savage, P.J., Sidney, S. and Wagenknecht, L.E. (1990). 'Obesity and overweight in young adults: The CARDIA study'. *Preventative Medicine*, 19:476-88

Cale, L. (2000). 'Physical activity promotion in secondary schools'. *European Physical Education Review*, 6:71-90

Cale, L. and Almond, L. (1992). 'Physical activity levels of young children: A review of the evidence'. *Health Education Journal*, 51:94-9

Carpenter, W.H., Poehlman, E.T., O'Connell, M. and Goran, M.I. (1995). 'Influence of body composition and resting metabolic rate on variation in total energy expenditure: A meta-analysis'. *American Journal of Clinical Nutrition*, 61:4–10

Caspersen, C.J., Powell, K.E. and Christenson, G.M. (1985). 'Physical activity, exercise and physical fitness: Definitions and distinctions for health-related research'. *Public Health Reports*, 100(2):126–31

Caterson, I.D. (1990). 'Management strategies for weight control: Eating, exertion and behaviour modification'. *Drugs*, 39(suppl.):20–32

Chief Medical Officer (CMO) (2002). 'Health Check: On the state of the public health – CMO's Annual Report 2002'. London, Department of Health (DH)

CMO (2000). 'Health Check: Obesity – defusing the health time-bomb – CMO's Annual Report 2002'. London, DH, 37–45

CMO (2004). 'At least 5 a week: Evidence on the impact of physical activity and its relationship to health'. London, DH

Cole, T.J. et al. (1995). 'Body mass index curves for the UK'. *Archives of Disease in Childhood*, 73:25–9

Corbin, C.B. and Fletcher, P. (1968). 'Diet and physical activity patterns of obese and non-obese elementary schoolchildren'. *Research Quarterly*, 39:922–8

Coulson, M. and Archer, D. (2008). *The Advanced Fitness Instructor's Handbook*. London, A&C Black

Coulson, M. and Archer, D. (2009). *Practical Fitness Testing*. London, A&C Black

Davison, K.K. and Birch, L.L. (2001). 'Weight status, parent reaction, and self-concept in five-year-old girls'. *Pediatrics*, 107:46–53

Deckelbaum, R.J. and Williams, C.L. (2001). 'Childhood obesity: The health issue'. *Obesity Research*, 9:S239–S243

Deitel, M. (2003). 'Overweight and obesity worldwide now estimated to involve 1.7 billion people'. *Obesity Surgery*, 13:329–330

Department for Culture Media and Sport (DCMS) & Strategy Unit (2002). 'Game Plan: A strategy for delivering the government's sport and physical activity objectives'. London, The Cabinet Office

Department for Education and Skills (DfES) (2007). 'Government Office Regions and LEAs'. UK, DfES ([Online] Available from: http://www.dfes.gov.uk/rsgateway/leas.shtml. [Accessed 12 March 2007])

Department for Education and the Welsh Office (1995). 'Physical Education and the National Curriculum'. London, Her Majesty's Stationery Office (HMSO)

Department of Health (DH) (1995). 'More People, More Active, More Often. Physical activity in England: A consultation paper'. London, HMSO

Devaney, B. and Stuart, E. (1998). 'Eating breakfast: Effects of the school programme'. Alexandria, VA, USDA Food and Nutrition Service

DH (2001). 'Health Survey for England: Avon longitudinal study of parents and children 1998. London, The Stationery Office (TSO)

DH (2003). 'Health Survey for England 2002: The health of children and young people'. London, TSO

DH (2004). 'Choosing Health: Making healthy choices easier'. London, TSO

DH (2005a). 'Choosing Health, Choosing Activity: A physical activity action plan'. London, DH

DH (2005b). 'Choosing Health, Choosing a Better Diet: A food and health action plan'. London, DH

DH (2005c). 'Delivering Choosing Health: Making healthier choices easier'. London, DH

DH (2006a). 'Choosing Health: Obesity Bulletin Issue 1'. London, DH

DH (2006b). 'Fact sheet on physical activity'. London, DH

DH (2006c). 'Health profile of England'. London, DH

DH (2006d). 'Measuring Childhood Obesity: Guidance to primary care trusts'. London, DH

DH (Joint Health Surveys Unit) (1999). 'Health Survey for England: Cardiovascular disease 1998'. London, TSO

DH and Sport England (SE) (2006). 'Local Exercise Action Pilots (LEAP): Summary of Interim Findings'. London, DH

Dietz, W.H. and Gortmaker, S.L. (1985). 'Do we fatten our children at the television set? Obesity and television viewing in children and adolescents'. *Pediatrics*, 75:807–12

Dietz, W.H., Bandini, L.G., Morelli, J.A., Peers, K.F. and Ching, P.L. (1994). 'Effect of sedentary activities on resting metabolic rate'. *American Journal of Clinical Nutrition*, 59:556–9

Duda, J.L. (2001). 'Achievement goal research in sport: Pushing the boundaries and clarifying some misunderstandings'. In G. C. Roberts (ed.), *Advances in Motivation in Sport and Exercise*. Champaign, Illinois, Human Kinetics, 129–82

Dyer, R. (1994). 'Traditional treatment of obesity: Does it work?' *Clinical Endocrinology Metabolism*, 8:661–88

Ekelund, U.M., Sjostrom, M., Yngve, A., Poortvliet, E., Nilsson, A., Froberg, K., Wederkopp, N. and Westerterp, K.R. (2001). 'Physical activity assessed by activity monitor and doubly labeled water in children'. *Medicine and Science in Sports and Exercise*, 33:275–81

Epstein, L.H., Wing, R.R., Koeske, R. and Valoski, A. (1984). 'Effects of diet plus exercise on weight changes in parents and children'. *Journal of Consultant Clinical Psychology*, 52:429–437

Epstein, L.H., Valoski, A., Wing, R.R. and McCurley, J. (1990). 'Ten-year follow-up of behavioural family based treatment for obese children'. *Journal of the American Medical Association*, 264:2519–23

Erikson, S.J., Robinson, T.N., Haydel, K.F. and Killen, J.D. (2000). 'Are overweight children unhappy? Body mass index, depressive symptoms, and overweight concerns in elementary school children'. *Archives of Pediatrics & Adolescent Medicine*, 154:931–5

Faigenbaum, A.D. and Avery, D. (1999). 'The effects of different resistance training protocols on muscular strength and endurance development in children', *Pediatrics*, 104(1):e5

Faigenbaum, A.D. and Avery, D. (2000). 'Strength training for children and adolescents'. *Clinical Sports Medicine*, 19(4):593–619

Fletcher, G.G., Balady, G., Blair, S.N., Blumenthal, J., Caspersen, C.J. and Chaitman, B. (1996). 'Statement on exercise: Benefits and recommendations for physical activity programs for all Americans. A statement for health professionals by the Committee on Exercise and Cardiac Rehabilitation of the Council on Clinical Cardiology, American Heart Association'. *Circulation*, 94:857–62

Fox, K.R. (2003). 'Childhood obesity and the role of physical activity'. *Journal of the Royal Society for the Promotion of Health*, 124(1):34–9

Gilliam, T.B., Freedson, P.S., Greener, D.L. and Shahraray, B. (1981). 'Physical activity patterns determined by heart rate monitoring in six 2–7 year old children'. *Medicine and Science in Sports and Exercise*, 13(1):65

Goran, M.I., Hunter, G., Nagy, T.R. and Johnson, R. (1997). 'Physical activity related energy expenditure and fat mass in young children'. *International Journal of Obesity*, 21:171–8

Gortmaker, S.L., Must, A., Perrin, J.M., Sobol, A.M. and Dietz, W.H. (1993). 'Social and economic consequences of overweight in adolescence and young adulthood'. *New England Journal of Medicine*, 329:1008–12

Graham, G., Holt/Hale, S. and Parker, M. (1993). *Children Moving: A Reflective Approach to Teaching Physical Education* (3rd edn). Mountain View, California, Mayfield

Gunnell, D.J., Frankel, S.J., Nanchahal, K., Peters, T.J. and Smith, G.D. (1998). 'Childhood obesity and adult cardiovascular mortality: A 57-year follow-up study based on the Boyd Orr cohort'. *American Journal of Clinical Nutrition*, 67:1111–18

Hall, D. and Elliman, D. (2003). *Health for All Children* (4th edn). Oxford Medical Publications, 184–8

Harris, J. (1994). 'Young people's perceptions of health, fitness and exercise: Implications for the teaching of health-related exercise'. *Physical Education Review*, 17(2):143–51

Harris, J. (1995). 'Physical education: A picture of health?' *British Journal of Physical Education*, 26(4):25–32

Harro, M. and Riddoch, C. (2000). 'Physical activity'. In N. Armstrong and W. van Mechelen (eds.), *Paediatric Exercise Science and Medicine*. Oxford, Oxford University Press, 77–82

Health Development Agency (2003). 'Evidence briefing: The management of obesity and overweight'. London, The Stationery Office (TSO)

Hill, A.J. (2005). 'Social and self-perception of obese children and adolescents'. In N. Cameron, N.G. Norgan and G.T.H. Ellison (eds.), *Childhood Obesity: Contemporary Issues*. Boca Raton, CRC Press, 39–49

Himes, J.H. and Dietz, W.H. (1994). 'Guidelines for overweight in adolescent preventive services: Recommendations from an expert committee'. *American Journal of Clinical Nutrition*, 59:307–16

Honeybourne, J., Hill, M. and Wyse, J. (1998). *PE for You*. Stanley Thornes, Cheltenham

Joint Health Surveys Unit (on behalf of the DH) (2003). 'Health Survey for England, 2002'. Norwich, The Stationery Office ([Online] Available from: www.doh.gov.uk/stats/trends1.htm)

Jumi, R.T. (1997). 'Obesity as a disease'. *British Medical Journal Bulletin*, 53:307–21

Ku, L.C., Shapiro, L.R., Crawford, P.B. and Huenemann, R.L. (1981). 'Body composition and physical activity in 8 year old children'. *American Journal of Clinical Nutrition*, 34:2270–75

Kuczmarski, R.J., Flegal, K.M., Campbell, S. and Johnson, C.L. (1994). 'Increasing prevalence of overweight among US adults: The National Health and Nutrition Examination Surveys, 1960–1991'. *Journal of the American Medical Association*, 272:205–11

Livingstone, M.B.E., Coward, W.A. and Prentice, A.M. (1992). 'Daily energy expenditure in free-living children: Comparison of heart rate monitoring with the doubly labelled water method'. *American Journal of Clinical Nutrition*, 56:343–52

Lytle, L. (2002). 'Nutritional issues for adolescents'. *Journal of the American Dietetic Association*, 102(3):8–13

McGill, H.C. (1984). 'Persistent problems in the pathogenesis of atherosclerosis'. *Arteriosclerosis*, 4:443–51

Mahan, L.K. (1987). 'Family-focused behavioural approach to weight control in children'. *Pediatric Clinician of North America*, 34:983–96

Matsudo, V.K.R., Matsudo, S. and Araujo, T. (1996). 'Relationship between physical fitness level at puberty and young adult life'. *Medicine and Science in Sports and Exercise*, 28:S23

Melanson, E.L. and Freedson, P.S. (1996). 'Physical activity assessment: A review of methods'. *Critical Reviews in Food Science and Nutrition*, 36:385–96

Melograno, V. (1979). *Designing curriculum and learning: A physical coeducation approach*. Dubuque, Iowa, Brown

Mossberg, H.O. (1989). '40-year follow-up of overweight children'. *The Lancet*, 2:491–3

Muecke, L., Simons-Morton, B. and Huang, I.W. (1992). 'Is childhood obesity associated with high fat foods and low physical activity?' *Journal of School Health*, 62:19–23

Must, A., Jaques, P.F., Dallal, G.E., Bajema, C.J. and Dietz, W.H. (1992). 'Long-term morbidity and mortality of adolescents: A follow up of the Harvard Growth Study of 1922–1935'. *New England Journal of Medicine*, 327:1350–55

National Audit Office (2001). 'Tackling Obesity in England: Report by the comptroller and auditor general'. London, TSO

National Institute for Health and Clinical Excellence (NICE) (2006). 'Obesity: the prevention, identification, assessment and management of overweight and obesity in adults and children'. London, NICE

National Institutes of Health (NIH) Consensus Development Panel on Physical Activity and Cardiovascular Health (1996). 'Physical activity and cardiovascular health'. *Journal of the American Medical Association*, 276:241–6

National Health Service (NHS) Centre for Reviews and Dissemination (1997). 'Systematic review of interventions in the treatment and prevention of obesity'. University of York, York Publishing Services

NHS (2006a). 'Statistics on Obesity, Physical Activity and Diet: England, 2006'. London, The Information Centre

NHS (2006b). 'The Health Survey for England 2005'. London, The information Centre ([Online] Available from http://www.ic.nhs.uk/pubs/hseupdate05 [Accessed: 31 March 2007])

Naughton, G., Farpour-Lambert, N.J., Carlson, J., Bradney, M. and Van Praagh, E. (2000). 'Physiological issues surrounding the performance of adolescent athletes'. *Sports Medicine*, 30(5):309–25

Obert, P., Mandigout, M., Vinet, A. and Courteix, D. (2001). 'Effect of a 13-week aerobic training programme on the maximal power developed during a force-velocity test in prepubertal boys and girls'. *International Journal of Sports Medicine*, 06:442–446

O'Conner, J. (2003). 'Measuring physical activity in children: A comparison of four different methods'. *Pediatric Exercise Science*, 15:202–15

Okasha, M. (2002). 'Body mass index in young adulthood and cancer mortality'. *Journal of Epidemiology and Community Health*, 56:780–4

Orbarzanek, E. (1994). 'Energy intake and physical activity in relation to indexes of body fat: The National Heart, Lung and Blood Institute Growth and Health Study'. *American Journal of Clinical Nutrition*, 60:15–22

Pate, R. R. (1993). 'Tracking of physical activity during early childhood'. *Medicine and Science in Sports and Exercise*, 25:S122

Pate, R.R., Freedson, P.S., Sallis, J.F., Taylor, W.C., Sirard, J., Trost, S.G. and Dowda, M. (2002). 'Compliance with physical activity guidelines: Prevalence in a population of children and youth'. *Annals of Epidemiology*, 12(5):303–8

Philip, W. (1997). 'Socioeconomic determinants of health'. *British Medical Journal*, 314:1545

Pitton, P.M. (1992). 'Prepubescent strength training: The effects of resistance training on strength gains in prepubescent children'. *National Strength and Conditioning Association Journal*, 14(6):55–7

Prentice, A.M. and Jebb, S.A. (1995). 'Obesity in Britain: Gluttony or sloth?' *British Medical Journal*, 311:437–9

Prochaska, J.O. and DiClemente, C.C. (1982). 'Transtheoretical therapy: Towards a more integrative model of change'. *Psychotherapy, Theory, Research and Practice*, 19(3):276–88

Prochaska, J.O., DiClemente, C.C. and Norcross, J.C. (1992). 'In search of how people change: Applications to addictive behaviours'. *The American Psychologist*, 47(9):1102–14

Reilly, J.J., Dorosty, A.R. and Emmett, P.M. (1999). 'Prevalence of overweight and obesity in British children: Cohort study'. *British Medical Journal*, 319(7216):1039

Reilly, J.J. and Dorosty, A.R. (1999). 'Epidemic of obesity in UK children'. *The Lancet*, 354(9193):1874–5

Richards, B.S. (1996). 'Slipped capital femoral epiphysis'. *Paediatric Reviews*, 17: 69–70

Riddoch, C.J. and Boreham, C.A. (1995). 'The health-related physical activity of children'. *Sports Medicine*, 19:86–102

Roberts, G.C. (1989). *Motivation in Sport and Exercise*. Champaign, Illinois, Human Kinetics, 273

Robinson, T.N. (1999). 'Reducing children's television viewing to prevent obesity: A randomised controlled trial'. *Journal of the American Medical Association*, 27(282):1561–7

Robinson, T.N., Hammer, L.D., Killen, J.D., Kraemer, H.C., Wilson, D.M., Hayward, C. and Taylor, C.B. (1993). 'Does television increase obesity and reduce physical activity? Cross sectional and longitudinal analysis among adolescent girls'. *Pediatrics*, 91:273–80

Rocchini, A.P., Katch, V., Anderson, J., Hinderliter, J., Becque, D., Martin, M. and Marks, C. (1988). 'Blood pressure in obese adolescents: Effect of weight loss'. *Pediatrics*, 82:16–23

Rowlands, A.V., Ingledew, D.K., Powell, S.M. and Eston, R.G. (1998). 'Validity of heart rate, pedometry, and accelerometry for predicting the energy cost of children's activities'. *Journal of Applied Physiology*, 84:362–71

Rowlands, A.V., Eston, R.G. and Ingledew, D.K. (1999). 'Relationship between activity levels, aerobic fitness, and body-fat in 8–10 year old children'. *Journal of Applied Physiology*, 86:1428–35

Rowlands, A.V., Eston, R.G. and Ingledew, D.K. (2000). 'The effect of type of physical activity measure on the relationship between body fatness and habitual physical activity in children: A meta-analysis'. *Annual of Human Biology*, 27:479–97

Sallis, J.F. (1993). 'Epidemiology of physical activity and fitness in children and adolescents'. *Critical Reviews in Food Science and Nutrition*, 33:403–8

Sallis, J.F. and Patrick, K. (1994). 'Physical activity guidelines for adolescents: A consensus statement'. *Pediatric Exercise Science*, 6:302–14

Sallis, J.F., Patterson, T. L., McKenzie, T. L. and Nader, P.R. (1988). 'Family variables and physical activity in preschool children'. *Journal of Deviant Behaviour in Pediatrics*, 9:57–61

Saris, W.H. (1986). 'Habitual physical activity in children: Methodology and findings in health and disease'. *Medicine and Science in Sports and Exercise*, 18:252–3

Sasaki, J., Shindo, M., Tanaka, H., Ando, M. and Arakawa, K. (1987). 'A long-term aerobic exercise program decreases the obesity index and increases the high density lipoprotein cholesterol concentration in obese children'. *International Journal of Obesity*, 11:339–45

Schmidt, R.A. (1988). *Motor Control and Learning: A Behavioral Emphasis* (2nd edn). Champaign, Illinois, Human Kinetics

Scottish Intercollegiate Guidelines Network (SIGN) (2003). 'Management of obesity in children and young people: A national clinical guideline'. Edinburgh, SIGN

SE (2004). 'The framework for sport in England: Making England an active and successful sporting nation, a vision for 2020'. London: Sport England ([Online] Available from: http://www.sportengland.org/national-framework-for-sport.pdf [Accessed 02.01.2007])

SE (2006). 'Sport England Annual Report and Accounts 2004–2005'. London, TSO

Serdula, M.K., Ivery, D., Coates, R.J., Freedman, D.S., Williamson, D.F. and Byers, T. (1993). 'Do obese children become obese adults? A review of the literature'. *Preventative Medicine*, 22:167–77

Siegel, J. (1988). 'Research Application: Fitness in prepubescent children: implications for exercise training'. *National Strength & Conditioning Association Journal*, 10(3):43–51

Simons-Morton, B.G., Parcel, G.S., O'Hara, N.M., Blair, S.N. and Pate, R.R. (1998). 'Health-related fitness in childhood: Status and recommendations'. *Annual Review of Public Health*, 9:403–25

Sleap, M. and Warburton, P. (1996). 'Physical activity levels of 5–11 year old children in England: Cumulative evidence from three direct observation studies'. *International Journal of Sports Medicine*, 17(4):248–53

Speednet (1999). 'Effects of the Suspension of the Order for National Curriculum Physical Education at Key Stages 1 and 2 on Physical Education in Primary Schools during 1989'. *Interim Summary of Findings. National 'Speednet' Survey*. Press Release, 19 Aug.

Stratton, G., Jones, M., Fox, K.R., Tolfrey, K., Harris, J., Maffulli, N., Lee, M. and Frustich,

S.P. (2004). BASES Position Statement on Guidelines for Resistence Exercise in Young People. *Journal of Sports Sciences*, 22(4):383–390

Strauss, R.S. (2000). 'Childhood obesity and self-esteem'. *Pediatrics*, 105:15

Sunnegardh, J., Bratteby, L.E., Hagman, U., Samuelson, G. and Sjolin, S. (1986). 'Physical activity in relation to energy intake and body fat in 8 and 13 year old children in Sweden'. *Acta Paediatrica Scandinavica*, 75:955–63

Suter, E. and Hawes, M.R. (1993). 'Relationship of physical activity, body fat, diet, and blood lipid profile in youths 10–15 years'. *Medicine and Science in Sports and Exercise*, 25:748–54

The Stationary Office. *Every Child Matters* (2004). Norwich

Treiber, F.A., Musante, L., Hartdagan, S., Davis, H., Levy, M. and Strong, W.B. (1989). 'Validation of a heart rate monitor for children in laboratory and field settings'. *Medicine and Science in Sports and Exercise*, 21:338–42

Troiano, R.P., Flegal, K.M., Kuczmarski, R.J., Campbell, S.M. and Johnson, C.L. (1995). 'Overweight prevalence and trends for children and adolescents: The National Health and Nutritional Examination Surveys, 1963–1991'. *Archives of Pediatrics & Adolescent Medicine*, 149:1085–91

Trost, S.G., Ward, D.S., Moorehead, S.M., Watson, P.D., Riner, W. and Burke, J.R. (1998). 'Validity of the computer science and applications (CSA) activity monitor in children'. *Medicine and Science in Sports and Exercise*, 30:629–33

Tucker, L.A. (1986). 'The relationship of television viewing to physical fitness and obesity'. *Adolescence*, 21:797–806

Wake, M., Hesketh, K. and Waters, E. (2003). 'Television, computer use and body mass index in Australian primary school children'. *Journal of Paediatrics and Child Health*, 39(2):130

Wallace, J.P., McKenzie, T. L. and Nader, P.R. (1985). 'Observed versus recalled exercise behaviour: A validation of a 7 day exercise recall for boys 11–13 years old'. *Research Quarterly for Exercise and Sport*, 56:161–5

Wanless, D. (2004). 'Securing Good Health for the Whole Population: Final Report'. London, HMSO

Welk, G.J., Corbin, C.B. and Dale, D. (2000). 'Measurement issues in the assessment of physical activity in children'. *Research Quarterly in Exercise and Sport*, 71:59–73

Welsman, J. and Armstrong, N. (2000). 'Physical activity patterns in secondary school children'. *European Journal of Physical Education*, 5:147–57

Wright, C.M., Parker, L., Lamont, D. and Craft, A.W. (2001). 'Implications of childhood obesity for adult health'. *British Medical Journal*, 323:1280–84

Yang, X., Telama, R. and Laakso, L. (1996). 'Parents' physical activity, socio-economic status and education as predictors of physical activity and sport among children and youths'. *International Review for Sociology of Sport*, 31(3):273–94

Index

Entries in italics are exercises. Page numbers in italics are illustrations. Page numbers with 't' are tables. These will appear when illustrations and tables are not within page ranges in the entries.